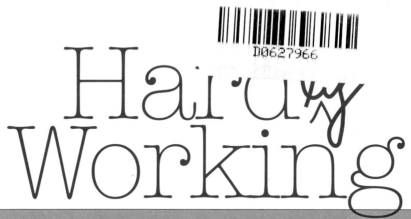

Hardly Working

The Overachieving Underperformer's Guide to Doing as Little as Possible in the Office

Written by Chris Morran
Illustrated by Mike Pisiak

SIMON SPOTLIGHT ENTERTAINMENT
New York   London   Toronto   Sydney

SIMON SPOTLIGHT ENTERTAINMENT
An imprint of Simon & Schuster
1230 Avenue of the Americas, New York, New York 10020

An EYE book

Conceived, designed, and produced by
EYE
276 Fifth Avenue
Suite 205
New York, NY 10001

Editorial and Art Direction: Michael Driscoll
Cover and Interior Design: Sheila Hart Design, Inc.
Copyeditor: Katherine Devendorf
Proofreader: Adam Sommers

Publisher: William Kiester

Manufactured in China
First Edition 10 9 8 7 6 5 4 3 2 1

Library of Congress Cataloging-in-Publication Data
Morran, Chris.
Hardly working / by Chris Morran ; illustrated by Mike Pisiak.
p. cm.
ISBN 0-689-87477-4
1. Work—Humor. 2. Business—Humor. I. Title.
PN6231.W644M67 2004
818'.602—dc22
2004011947

Acknowledgments and Dedication

Because I can barely tie my shoes without assistance, acknowledgments are due to the following: William Kiester and Michael Driscoll at EYE; Kim Tracey, Marthas Mihalick and McCool, and Emily Russo; Chris Garcia, Kevin and Kelly Finn, and Jessica Anderson; and the good people at O'Connor's. Thanks also to Mike Pisiak for his spot-on illustrations, Sheila Hart for her wonderful design, and my publishers for the opportunity.

For my mother, Margaret, who knows all too well the inside of a cubicle. And for my nieces and nephew, may they never have the displeasure.

Contents

Introduction 7

I: Johnny-Come-Lately: Getting In Late

1. Always Be Prepared:
Setting Up the Right Props the Night Before 11
2. The Telltale Bag/Briefcase and What to Do with It. . . 16
3. Fast Food Is Good Food 19
4. A Little Morning Music Makes All the Difference. . . . 22
TRICKS OF THE TRADE: The Beauty of Voice Mail,
aka the Three Cs 27
5. The Early Bird Doesn't Just Get the Worm,
He Gets to Go Home Before Everyone Else. 30
6. Looking the Part: How to Appear Like You're
Not Just Getting In to the Office. 33
TRICKS OF THE TRADE: Getting Away with It:
Your Guide to Office Excuses 38

II: The Longer Lunch: The Tray of Half-Eaten Food and Other Time-Wasting Methods

7. Lovely Leftovers: Salvation in a Paper Sack 47
8. Acting 101: How to Look Like You're Working
Through Lunch While Writing Your Novel 51
TRICKS OF THE TRADE: Planning Carl's Birthday Party:
A Timeline of a Perfectly Wasted Day 56
9. Dine & Dash: The Culinary Art of Deception 58
10. The "Interview" and Other Ways to Get
Your Coworkers to Cover for You. 63
TRICKS OF THE TRADE: From Clark Kent to Superman:
Tips for Changing Into Your Interview Clothes
Without Arousing Suspicion 67

III: Looking Busy While Doing Nothing

11 Clutter Is Beautiful:
Simple Steps to a Busy-Looking Office 71
12 Behind Closed Doors: Getting People to Leave You Alone . 77
13 Identifying and Dealing With Snooping Coworkers 81
14 The "Big Project": Exploiting Massive Corporate
Bureaucracies for Your Benefit 85
TRICKS OF THE TRADE: Tetris, Minesweeper,
and Solitaire (aka The Trinity) 89
15 Billy Has Two Bosses:
Playing Your Superiors Against Each Other 93
16 Exploiting the "Home Office" and Other Corporate
Bogeymen to Get Others to Do Your Work 98
17 Grassroots Complaining:
The Tactical Distribution of Bitching and Moaning . . 101
18 Quid Pro Quo: Identifying Other Overachieving
Underperformers and Methods of Mutual Back Scratching . 107
19 Hide-and-Go-Sleep: Securing Nap Zones Within the Office . 112
20 Burning the Midnight Oil: The Late Stayer 119
TRICKS OF THE TRADE: The Shut Door and Tape Recorder. 123

IV: It's Nice to Be the Boss: Using Your Assistant to Do Even Less

21 Judging the Poker Face: Hints on Hiring 127
22 Follow My Lead: The Coattails Effect 131
23 "He's in a Meeting," or the Human "Do Not Disturb" Sign . 134
24 "Hold My Calls," or the Human Answering Machine . . . 139
TRICKS OF THE TRADE: Interns:
The Best Things in Life Are Free 142
25 When the Cat's Away: Making Your Assistant Glad
That You're Out of the Office 144
26 Need-to-Know: Why You Should Never
Tell Your Assistant the Whole Truth 148
27 A Rolling Assistant Gathers No Moss:
Why It's Good to Have Your Assistant Running Errands. 151
TRICKS OF THE TRADE: Giving Out Gold Stars:
Cheap Ways to Make Your Staff Happy 156

Afterword. 159

You're doing it again. You know you shouldn't, but some inexorable force compels you, and so you sink further into the abyss. It's killing you, gnawing away at what remains of your spent body, day after day. You rationalize the problem, telling yourself that everyone else does it, that it doesn't have you in its claws. Of course, you could just suck it up and go cold turkey, but you've heard tell of the horrors that decision has wrought upon others. And so you wake up and you do it again: You go to work.

Wouldn't it be amazing not to fear your morning commute? To find employment so thrilling and rewarding that the mere notion of going to the office propelled you out of bed in the morning, eager to face the day? Unfortunately the dreary reality of the situation is that most of us start the workday already counting down the nanoseconds until its conclusion. And though many office workers each face the same daily irritations (mountains of mind-numbing work with no real purpose, bosses who can't remember your name but who always catch you on a personal phone call, endless memos from nameless executives), the particular methods for coping with these miseries vary wildly. The **Overachiever**, for example, views this rote cycle as a challenge and arrives at his desk early, eager to show his boss just how well he can do his job. Bosses like these people. Conversely, the **Underperformer** quite obviously loathes his daily ordeal and lopes into the office late, his dread at being required to perform his tasks becoming greater and more apparent by the day. Bosses fire these people. Straddling the line, the **Overachieving Underperformer** comes and goes at will but manages to appear at all times to be working hard. Bosses love these people, but only because they don't know any better.

The Overachiever

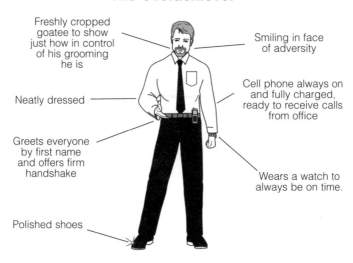

Freshly cropped goatee to show just how in control of his grooming he is

Smiling in face of adversity

Cell phone always on and fully charged, ready to receive calls from office

Neatly dressed

Greets everyone by first name and offers firm handshake

Wears a watch to always be on time.

Polished shoes

The Underperformer

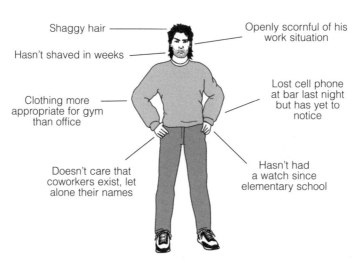

Shaggy hair

Openly scornful of his work situation

Hasn't shaved in weeks

Lost cell phone at bar last night but has yet to notice

Clothing more appropriate for gym than office

Doesn't care that coworkers exist, let alone their names

Hasn't had a watch since elementary school

The Overachieving Underperformer

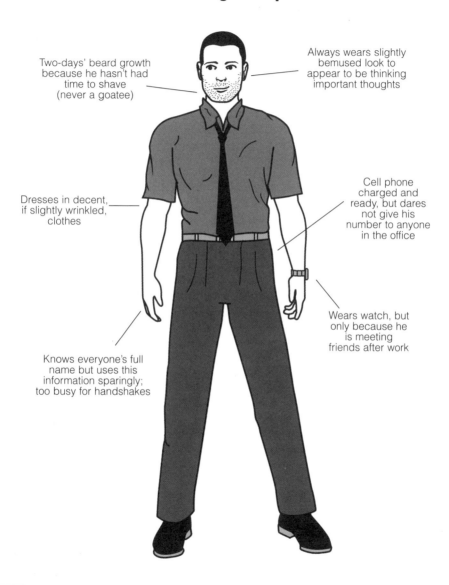

Two-days' beard growth because he hasn't had time to shave (never a goatee)

Always wears slightly bemused look to appear to be thinking important thoughts

Dresses in decent, if slightly wrinkled, clothes

Cell phone charged and ready, but dares not give his number to anyone in the office

Knows everyone's full name but uses this information sparingly; too busy for handshakes

Wears watch, but only because he is meeting friends after work

Section I
Johnny-Come-Lately:
Getting In Late

For some cruel reason, most offices require their employees to be at work and raring to make themselves useful at a dreadfully early hour. For most people, needing to get to work on time is an immutable fact, and they plan their mornings accordingly. To a small group of Early Birds (See Chapter 5), arriving shortly after the crack of dawn is actually preferred. But for the great majority, there's an evil subtext to the letters "A.M." Since simply sleeping in and hoping no one notices your absence is not an option (lest you plan on filing for unemployment when you wake up), you'll need to be well versed in the fine art of concealing tardiness.

Chapter 1

Always Be Prepared:
Setting Up the Right Props the Night Before

It's Wednesday morning. The shrill scream of your alarm clock has rudely rousted you from your bed. You have twenty minutes to clean yourself up, get dressed, and cover the thirty-minute commute to your office. Simply put, there is no possible way that you will make it to work on time this morning.

But the Overachieving Underperformer (OU) doesn't need to worry. Why? Because he took five minutes at the end of the previous workday to see to a few simple precautions that will save him his job and still give him time to enjoy a decent shower.

1   **The Conspicuous Coat**

Treat yourself. Go out and purchase a new coat, one that's a bit brighter than what you'd normally wear, but nothing too garish. Wear it out every day to lunch, or whenever you leave to run a work-related errand (which is often). When you're not wearing the coat, drape it over the back of a chair in your office where anyone can see it.

What people don't know is that, except during the aforementioned lunches and errands, that coat never leaves the office. At the end of every day while you head home, the coat remains behind, clearly visible to passing eyes. And in the morning when you're still at home shaking off the sleepies, the coat is hard at work, letting people assume that you are too—you must be around the office somewhere, just briefly away from your desk. Meanwhile you're sitting on the couch catching the end of your favorite morning talk show.

2   **Job Saver**

A skilled Overachieving Underperformer knows never to turn off the computer; there are fewer things that signal "NOT IN YET!!" than a dark monitor. And only slightly less deadly is having a screen saver running. Sure, you could easily turn off your screen saver and leave the monitor running all night, which would fend off the casual passerby. But if someone comes by looking for you several times and sees the same, unchanged image on your computer, it might arouse suspicion.

Instead, you need to take technology's negatives and turn them to your advantage. Make a handful of screen captures of various spreadsheets, memos, and e-mails. Then take these images and put them into a very slow rotation as your screen saver. Even if someone makes repeat visits to your desk in the morning, it will appear that you've been there in the interim. In the meantime take the scenic route to work, the one that passes through the local diner and comes with a side order of hash browns.

3 Cleaning Up

So long as you're able to convince them not to touch the mess on your desk (see Chapter 11 for more on clutter) or hang up that coat you're always absentmindedly leaving behind, you shouldn't have any problems with the cleaning staff that comes in every night to sweep and vacuum. But there is one other threat that custodians pose, and it's a potentially fatal one: They always turn out the lights when they're done.

So that this doesn't foil your plans the next time you sense a late morning coming on, take a moment the night before to chat with the staff member assigned to your hallway. Tell him or her that you are only going out for a few hours, and that you'd like it very much if your light was left on. Confide that you have an irrational fear of burglars and the glow of the fluorescent lights comforts you. This will ensure that your light shines through the night—and is still on when others arrive in the morning.

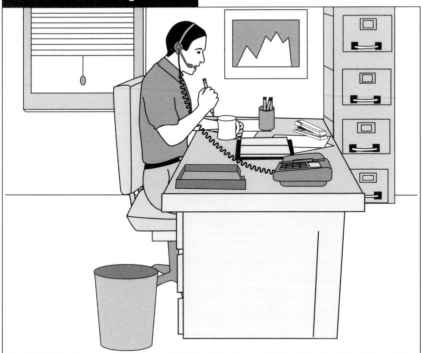

But what if it comes time to make your exit and the cleaning crew is nowhere to be found? (Maybe they've got some work-avoidance tricks of their own.) If you're unable to ensure that your light will shine all night, wait until just before you go to bed, then leave a message for that coworker (let's call her Tricia) who's always the first one in the office. Fill Tricia's voice mail with a long, anxious message about how you think you've lost your wallet, and how

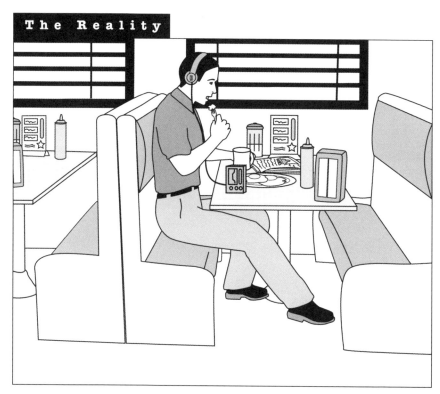

you wonder if she might look under your desk as soon as she gets in. Tricia, being a decent person, will go into your office, turn on the light, and move your chair away from the desk. Voilà! She has just unwittingly clocked you in. When you enter undetected forty-five minutes late, be sure to give Tricia one of the doughnuts you picked up on the way to work.

Chapter 2

The Telltale Bag/Briefcase
and What to Do with It

One thing you've got to ask yourself as you broaden your Overachieving Underperformer's repertoire is this: How necessary is your handbag and/or briefcase? Really, in this time of the almost all-digital workplace, how much are you actually carting back and forth from the office? If you're an early-rising nonworker (see Chapter 5), you could make the argument that the image of you lugging a cumbersome bag around only adds to the general, misguided impression that you are a diligent employee. But for those of us who need to enter the office without turning heads, being seen carrying any sort of bag paints us as the idle people we pretend not to be. However, if you absolutely must bring a bag or a briefcase (perhaps you've got some magazines you'd like to read while you're faking work?), there are some options.

1 Ditch It ASAP

You can always go back and get it later. If you drive to work, leave it in the car. If you have essential papers or files that you need in order to do your pretend job, put them in a folder and take them with you. For some reason, being seen with a briefcase makes you look guilty, whereas being seen carrying a stack of papers makes you look busy.

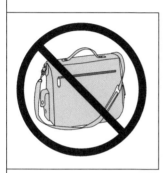

For those who don't drive to work, things are trickier. If your office has a front reception or security desk and you are friendly with the people there, leave your bag with them, saying, "A friend will be by in a couple of hours to pick this up." If you have to, leave a fake note for your imaginary friend. Once you've settled in to the office and are out of the danger zone, go back and retrieve your items, blaming your flaky friend for changing his mind.

2 The Stone-Faced Lie

Should you find yourself unable to stash your bag before entering the office proper and are spotted by the boss with your bag in hand, you'll need to attempt a potentially risky maneuver: Claim that you've got a loose filling and your dentist was only able to squeeze you in at ten a.m. And since you weren't sure how long you'd be away from the office, you came in early to get some work done. So long as you don't falter in your excuse-making, your boss should let you off with nothing more than a "You should really tell me before you leave for an appointment" scolding. And in just a matter of seconds you've turned a nearly fatal faux pas into another two hours of free time that morning.

Overachieving at Underperforming

If you're someone who can get through the day without toting around any sort of bag, there's an opportunity to use that to your advantage. Much like the coat fake-out in Chapter 1, this trick involves a bag that never leaves the office, but it differs from the coat deception in the placement. Whereas the coat is something intended to be seen by all, the bag should be situated in a place where it would only be discovered upon closer inspection. Leaving the bag sitting by the side of your desk or hanging from a coat hook are nice options.

Additionally, certain accoutrements can help give the illusion that this bag is not something left behind at the end of the day—an old cellular phone that you don't use anymore (or a convincing toy facsimile) sticking out of a side pocket, a scarf draped over the shoulder strap in the winter, an umbrella in the spring. Use your imagination!

Chapter 3

Fast Food
Is Good Food

There are those people who will tell you that the most important part of a balanced diet is partaking of a healthy, nutritious breakfast—that doughnuts, pastries, bacon, and other vilified morning staples only serve to slow you down. Although they may have all sorts of numbers and scientific data backing their statements, they lack the vision of the Overachieving Underperformer. Where nutritionists and dieticians see useless calories and fat, we recognize an invaluable resource that will aid us in avoiding large chunks of work in the morning hours.

1 Feed, Forgive, and Forget

For those mornings when you're running late but were unable to adequately prepare the night before, you need to transition from sneak-attack mode into a damage-control position. In such situations, bribery is always a good idea. And for most people, food is second only to cash in its ability to sway their opinion.

Since you're already destined to arrive after everyone else, it can't hurt to stop by your local doughnut shop and stock up. Make sure to score an array of treats for your coworkers; it helps to know the snack preferences of your boss, and of those coworkers who are most critical of other employees whom they perceive as not doing their fair share of the work. It's very hard to be upset with someone who not only knows that you salivate over lemon tarts, but also actually goes out of her way to make sure there's one in the bag for you.

Sure, some people may see through your thinly veiled attempt to curry your coworkers' and boss's favor, but their complaints will fall upon the deaf ears of coworkers swept up in the sugar high. Within a matter of minutes you will have transformed yourself from a lazy oversleeper into a thoughtful and generous part of the staff.

2 Being the Good Gofer

Imagine the following scenario: You're late, but you've managed to enter the building unseen. And then, just as you arrive at your desk and begin taking off your jacket, you look up to see the boss standing in your office doorway. How do you get yourself out of this particular squeeze?

First you must remember that while, yes, the boss is glaring suspiciously in your direction, you are not caught yet. If you take stock of the scene and don't panic, this potential embarrassment could actually end up working to your advantage. If she's suddenly come upon you in the middle of the settling-in process, there's still an out.

She doesn't know whether you're in the middle of putting the jacket on or taking it off, so play into that uncertainty and start slipping your arms back into the sleeves. Unless she's completely oblivious she'll ask where you think you're going. Acting surprised by her query, assure her that you're feeling really sluggish after reviewing files all morning and are running to get some coffee, maybe a Danish. Then, as if you're sorry you hadn't thought of it earlier, ask her if she'd like anything while you're out. If she says no, be amiably insistent: "C'mon, my treat!" In the worst possible situation, she takes you up on the generous offer and you're out a few dollars. Regardless of what your boss decides to do, you've just converted a scenario in which a scolding would be appropriate into a twenty-minute trip to the doughnut shop.

Chapter 4

A Little Morning Music
Makes All the Difference

As you've already seen, it's to your advantage to go to every possible length to make your coworkers and superiors believe that you're already in the office when they arrive in the morning. To that end, something as simple as a clock radio can be your salvation, filling your office with the music of believability. If used incorrectly, however, that same radio could be broadcasting the sounds of your doom.

There are several important factors involved in selecting your ideal audio setup, from the type of radio to the genre of music, from how early you set the timer to how loud you set the volume. Consider carefully the following, and decide on the options that are best suited to your idleness.

Types of Radio

 CD Player

Pros:

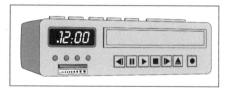

- Prerecorded CDs allow for more control over the content of what plays while you're not in the office. You can carefully plan your music choices to create a desired impression.
- CD listeners give off the air of being more focused, controlled people, not wanting to be distracted by the randomness and commercial interruption of a radio broadcast.

Cons:

- CDs have limited playing times, usually around forty-five minutes. If you don't arrive in time to change the CD, your office will be plagued with dead air until you get there.
- Being somewhat fragile objects, CDs do occasionally skip or get stuck in one spot. If this should happen in your absence, others will most certainly notice.

2 **AM/FM Radio**

Pros:

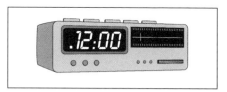

- Any clock radio can be set to play at a given time every morning.
- Variety: Because of the nature of live radio, a station will not broadcast the same playlist every morning.

Cons:

- Clock radios are not well regarded for their clear,

dependable reception. You run the risk of having the radio blaring fuzzy voices or static all morning.

- Some employers look down upon listening to the radio at work, considering it a distraction on par with reading the newspaper or browsing the Web.

Types of Music

Analyzing the positives and negatives of each of the thousands of recognized genres of music would require several volumes. And that would require work. Thus, it's most efficient to deal with only a few general types.

Overachieving at Underperforming

Knowing your boss's particular tastes in music, then mimicking them, can be extremely helpful. People in authority like to believe that those under their supervision aspire to become them. If you can, feed into your boss's ego and be his musical mirror.

 Classical

There are many forms of what is referred to as classical music, but to most people the term implies strings, pianos, and the occasional French horn. Whether or not there is any truth to the argument, almost everyone has heard about studies showing that listening to classical music improves concentration. At the very least, the mere sound of an orchestra playing on your office radio gives your coworkers the idea that you've got a sensitive, bookish side—and that you're less likely to be taking a nap in the backseat of your car. On the other hand, there's the possibility of having to fake your way through a conversation with a boss or coworker who actually knows something about classical music. It's one thing to pretend to listen to a concerto, another to actually know what a concerto is. Should someone attempt to engage you in a detailed conversation about the Budapest Philharmonic's "Fugue in B-Sharp" or some such, play the blissful ignorance card: "I don't know a lot about classical music. All I know is that it relaxes me ... and that Yo-Yo Ma really can play."

2 Easy Listening

As a category this one is pretty self-explanatory: non-offensive, quiet to mid-volume tunes. Leaving aside any discussion of artistic merit, such music is generally a safe bet for convincing people that you're around in the morning. Even if you're not known as a soft-music sort of person by your coworkers, it's believable that you'd choose to listen to something milder in the morning—especially since you're getting in to the office so early!

3 Pop/Rock

Here you're looking at music from the mid-Sixties to the present that can range from bubblegum pop to guitar-driven rock. However, this is a category including only the most popular of these tunes; no boundary-pushing here. This is music that everyone knows, simply because of its pervasiveness. Played at a barely audible volume, anyone passing by your work space will assume that you're in the office and just away from your desk.

WARNING: Don't play this music too loud, as you'll run the risk of broadcasting a catchy tune that could inadvertently draw others into your area.

4 **Niche Genres**

This is the riskiest of all the types of music. Bands that fall within specific genre categories tend to have divisive effects on new listeners. On one hand, your boss could walk by your office, hear your favorite CD playing, not like it, and decide that you're not his type of person. Conversely, your boss could be intrigued by what he hears, which may compel him to pull out the CD to see for himself what you're listening to—or worse yet, he could stand around waiting for you to get back to your desk. So while the boss might like your music, he might fire you for being late to work.

The Beauty of Voice Mail, aka the Three Cs

The advent of voice mail systems that allow you to check and send messages from remote locations has revolutionized life for the Overachieving Underperformer. Not only do they allow you to dodge unwanted phone calls, but also in the hands of the right person they can be utilized to create the illusion of being a decent and punctual employee, despite constant oversleeping. To maximize voice mail's full job-retaining potential, one must learn, love, and live the **Three Cs.**

1. **CHANGING** the date on your outgoing voice mail message. Yes, it's annoying and it eats up thirty seconds of your time that might be better spent doing nothing; but if you can find it within yourself to become one of those people who change the date on their outgoing voice mail message daily—especially if you do it the night before—the positive results are twofold. First, it takes advantage of the public's misguided notion that anyone fastidious enough to record a new voice mail message every day is a good and detail-oriented employee. You're giving the appearance of being on top of things, when really all you're doing is looking at a calendar and reciting the date. Second, by changing the message at the end of every workday, you've preemptively got your butt covered for your inevitable late arrival the next morning. It's widely accepted that most voice mail date-changers go through this daily routine first thing in the morning. But by having done this the

night before, you've bought yourself a fifteen-minute arrival bumper. Anyone trying to reach you will hear your already-updated message and assume you're in and just busy.

2 CHECKING your voice mails before you arrive at the office. This is a prime example of dressing yourself up in the trappings of a responsible employee in order to

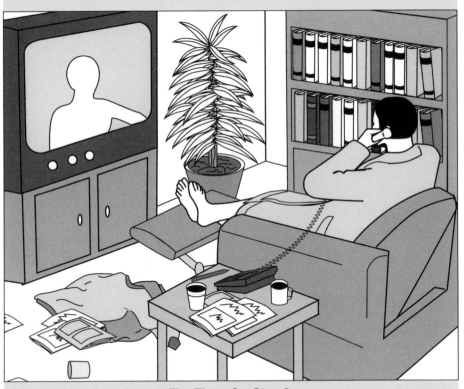

The Three Cs, Step 2:
Checking your voice mail before you arrive

ultimately act irresponsibly, in this case by showing up late. Calling from home or your cell phone to check any messages that already have been left allows you to defuse any potentially explosive situations that might arise by your slinking in forty minutes after everyone else. It's one thing to arrive late and oblivious. It's another to show up knowing the situation and pretending to care.

3 **CHOOSING** whom to leave early-morning messages for. Almost all networked voice mail systems allow you to record a message and then send it on to another networked voice mail box. If you can prerecord messages and choose to have them sent at a later, scheduled time, that's fantastic. But most people will have to suffice with calling either before you leave in the morning or from the road. Select from your group of coworkers either the very gullible, the very hard of hearing, or the very busy. Leave a vague message about something or other. (If there's nothing real to discuss, make something up.) These people will believe you're calling from the office, will be unable to tell that you're calling from a cell phone, or (best of all) may just erase your message before it's finished. Regardless, they all now think that you are in the office when, in fact, you're taking the scenic route to work. And should your boss accuse you of tardiness, you've got ear-witness testimony to your having been in the office all morning.

Chapter 5

The Early Bird Doesn't Just Get the Worm, He Gets to Go Home Before Everyone Else

It's a widely held misconception, both in the business world and in the world at large, that early risers are harder working, more productive citizens. But the truth is that there are multitudes of dawn greeters as slothful and idle as any oversleeper. However, by virtue of being awake before some people even go to bed, these Early Birds are summarily held in higher regard than the typical Overachieving Underperformer. Thus, depending on your particular loafing desires, it may be to your advantage to occasionally set the alarm clock an hour earlier. If you find yourself in the enviable situation of being both lazy and up before sunrise, here are some tips on how to exploit people's preconceptions so you can spend those morning hours as idly as you wish.

First, you've got to be aware of *what* time your boss or bosses arrive in the morning, and then learn to be there immediately before they step through the door. So long as you're in the office first, who's to say what time you started working. Suppose, for example, you get to your desk at seven thirty and the boss saunters in at seven thirty-five. Unless you're required by some whip-wielding-supervisor to clock in every morning, there is nothing keeping your boss from believing that you've already been at your desk, toiling away, for hours.

Another advantage Early Birds have over everyone else is that they enjoy much more leeway when it comes to doing things that other employees would be frowned upon for doing. For instance, if you're in before everyone else, it's perfectly acceptable to take a little break to go out and pick up some morning munchies; after all, you did skip breakfast, and you were in an hour before the rest of your coworkers, right? Of course, in order to maximize your time, wait until others have begun to arrive before making a food run. It would just be wasted time-wasting if no one is there to see how hard you're pretending to work.

The early morning also allows for longer lingering around the coffee machine and lengthy, relaxing trips to the bathroom. (Bring a newspaper to read; you've got the time.) If you go so far as to deign to make the first pot of coffee for your coworkers, or perform some other ridiculously easy task like turning on lights, your colleagues not only will appreciate you and think of you as an essential member of the staff, but also they'll be much more forgiving of your sundry other shortcomings.

Of course, the best part of getting in to the office first is getting out of the office first. While all your coworkers drag themselves through that last hour of work, you're getting a jumpstart on the commute. Even better, for those nights when you pretend to work normal hours (or—say it ain't so—work late), everyone's view of your work ethic will increase exponentially. Of course, they don't know that you're only feigning a heavy workload while killing time until your dinner date or the ball game. By simply loitering in your office for an extra hour, you're passively earning brownie points toward promotions and bonuses.

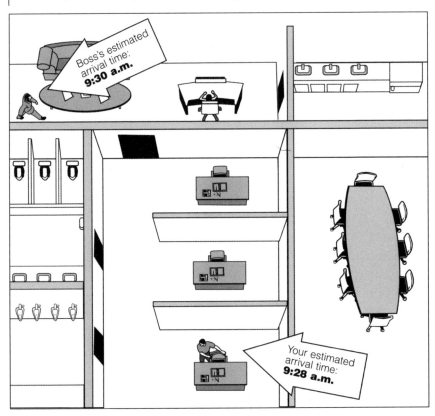

Chapter 6

Looking the Part: How to Appear Like You're Not Just Getting In to the Office

One of the keys to success as an Overachieving Underperformer is attention to detail—not the details of the work you're not doing, but the physical giveaways that suspicious bosses and coworkers might pick up on. These hypercritical types are fully aware that someone who's just getting in to work an hour late has a different appearance from the people who've already been at their desks working. They know the signals to watch out for, and if you're ever to defeat these people, you must know them, too. Let's examine the just-arrived worker from head to foot.

1 Hat Hair

It happens to us all, especially during the winter months when a heavy wool cap is all that stands between you and hypothermia. You finally get to work and take off the hat, only to have people gawking and giggling at your mussed and matted mop. It's usually several minutes before you realize that your hair is beaten down and disheveled. You've got a horrible case of hat hair. However, by the time you get to work, everyone else has corrected his or her tonsorial troubles and you stick out like a tousled troublemaker. What to do?

The easiest solution is obvious: Go right to the bathroom and fix the mess. But there is always peril in such situations, never knowing just whom you'll run into in the lavatory. You're less at risk if your office has small, single-occupancy bathrooms or if you work in a massive corporate complex where you can safely use a bathroom in a department where you'll be unrecognized.

The advanced Overachieving Underperformer, however, will play against people's preconceptions and exploit having the benefit of the doubt. Don't fix your hair; in fact, don't take off the hat. Leave it on and wear it all day. Or take it off at random times throughout the day and put it back on when least expected. People won't know whether you're coming or going and will eventually not give any thought to the hat or the bad hair hidden beneath. You've just taken away a weapon of the eagle-eyed boss out to ensnare latecomers.

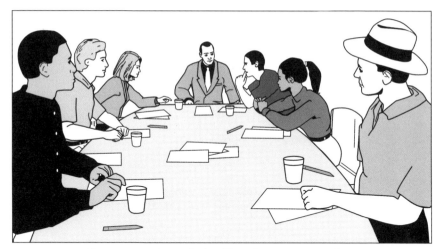

**Always wearing a hat will make your coworkers
think you're eccentric. Only you will know it's to cover up
the hat hair from your arrival fifteen minutes earlier.**

2 Layers, Layers, Layers

Jackets, scarves, gloves, and other such outerwear should be dealt with in much the same way as handbags, shoulder bags, and briefcases, discussed in Chapter 2. Basically, if you can leave them in the car or stash them somewhere away from your desk, then do so. And if you are able to go sans jacket to and from work, even better. There are also a few positive things to be said for wearing several layers instead of just one heavy coat. For instance, you may want to try wearing four layers (undershirt, cotton button-down, sweater, zip-up sweatshirt) that are appropriate both indoors and out, instead of dealing with a bulky, hard-to-hide winter jacket. Again, by not giving your

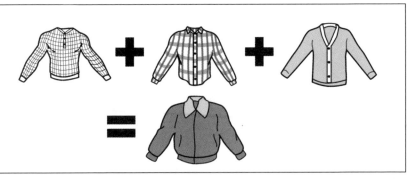

**Layers can replace a bulky coat—
a dead giveaway to the fact that you're just arriving.**

boss any definite signal stating "I just got into work! Please fire me," you're protecting your job and ensuring another paycheck.

3 **Not So Neat!**

It may seem counterintuitive to say that looking too neat in the morning marks you as a latecomer, but it is the truth. This is especially the case for coat-and-tie corporate jobs where almost every suit that comes through the door is freshly pressed and crisp and every tie is knotted with care. An hour or two of hard work will inevitably soften those pleats and loosen the necktie a notch. And since you want to look like one of these people without having to do any of the accompanying work, you've got to put some thought into your costume.

Tuck in your shirt so it's nice and stiff, and then do a couple of jumping jacks to simulate an hour's worth of moving about the office. Slide that tie on like a good junior executive, and then run your finger around the collar a few times to loosen it just so. Roll the sleeves up and down a few times, like you've been dealing intently with some tense situation. Pay attention to the people in your office who actually do a lot of work and follow their lead (in how to dress, not with regard to your career). If you pull this off successfully, your superiors will simply assume that you're a young go-getter just like the coworkers you're aping.

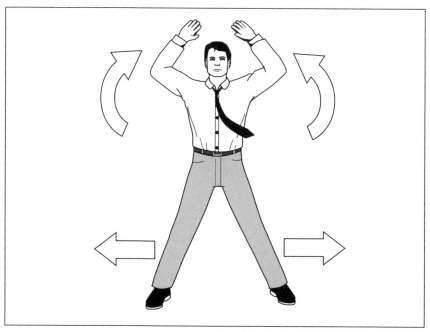

A quick set of jumping jacks in your office
will give your clothes the ruffled appearance
of someone who's already been working for an hour.

Tricks of the Trade

Getting Away with It:
Your Guide to Office Excuses

Unless you have a clueless supervisor who cares little about attendance in the workplace, getting some quality time away from the office demands a quality excuse. As a general rule, slipping away early requires some sort of concrete, unchangeable commitment, while sneaking in late is best explained away in terms of being caught up in circumstances beyond your control. Here are the most common excuses for missing work, and some helpful hints for selecting the right one for the occasion.

 Birth in the Family

Example: "My sister had a baby last night and I need time off to go see her in the hospital."

Ideal usage: Taking a half-day to get outside and enjoy the weather. Remember, just because your sister is in the hospital with a new child doesn't mean you actually have to use your time off to visit her.

Duration: One day.

Note: Birth of twins generally good for an extra half-day.

Believability: If your coworkers are unfamiliar with your relations, it shouldn't be too hard to pull the wool over their eyes. But if anyone knows anything about your family, you're going to have a difficult time convincing the more skeptical elements.

Versatility: For the agile liar this excuse can be utilized at any time. For everyone else you'll have to wait until one of your family members is with child.

Backstory: People like hearing about babies so much that they'll want to see pictures. Be prepared for an onslaught of questions about the newborn; if you're not telling the truth, you'd better be an excellent liar. Come prepared with weight, height, and one eccentric detail for added realism. ("You can bet Dad was surprised when he got a look at those Asian features!")

Frequency: For obvious reasons this excuse is not to be used too frequently, and certainly no more than once every nine months per relative.

Pros: By showing your closeness to your family, you'll likely improve people's perceptions of you.

Cons: Lying about something like a baby is too fraught with traps for all but the ablest of storytellers, so this should really be used only if there's a degree of truth to what you're telling your boss.

2 ## Death in the Family

Example: "My great-uncle Cyrus passed away the other night and I would appreciate having the day off to mourn."

Ideal usage: Getting away for a day trip out of town.

Duration: One to three days.

Believability: You're solid. Unless you have a reputation for telling horrible untruths, only the most crass coworker will openly express skepticism.

Versatility: Given the high believability factor of this excuse, you can make use of the fake funeral at any time.

Backstory: Since you're mourning the death of a nonexistent distant relative, you can get away with answering any probing questions with a pinched face, a long pause, and a quiet "I really can't talk about it yet." Even so, it doesn't hurt to have a brief history at the ready. ("Uncle Cyrus met my

Aunt Ginnie on a shrimp boat in Mississippi ...")
Frequency: While not a tale to be overused—lest your human resources manager start requesting death certificates—the timely passing of a semi-distant, fictional relative is a dependable, once-a-year free pass for a day or three of lounging around the house in your pajamas.
Pros: Can easily be played to earn unmerited sympathy, possibly reducing your short-term workload; even though you only ask for the morning off, any decent boss will throw in the afternoon so as not to appear heartless.
Cons: You're inevitably going to have to deal with some well-meaning boss or coworker trying to make you feel better.

3 **Doctor's Appointment**
Example: "I've got a doctor's appointment at two thirty; I should be back by four."
Ideal usage: Getting away for a job interview or checking out an afternoon ball game.
Duration: Two to six hours (one day maximum).
Believability: So common as to generally go unquestioned. Perhaps the quintessential "I'm leaving the office for a few hours and there's nothing you can do about it" excuse.
Versatility: Flexible. Operates equally well for preplanned half-days and spur-of-the-moment "I need to get out of here now" decisions. Although the doctor's appointment is generally only good for half a day, you can choose whether you want to come in late or leave early.
Backstory: If used infrequently, you can get away with meaningless reasons like "My back is a little sore" or "I have this cold that I can't shake." Frequent employment of this excuse requires more elaborate evasions. (You may want to stock up on some medical textbooks.)

Note: If you're willing to go the extra mile, keep a plastic bag holding a new toothbrush and a roll of dental floss in your desk. It's a nice touch when returning from an alleged dental appointment, just as a pair of throwaway sunglasses will really help sell that visit to the optometrist.

Frequency: Three to five times per year is acceptable for general health maintenance. Those bold enough to latch on to a lingering malady (shingles, multiple wart removal, etc.) could theoretically utilize this excuse as often as once a week, and for an indefinite period of time.

Pros: By making the offer to return from the "appointment" before the day's end, you almost guarantee that your boss will give you the rest of the day free.

Note: If your boss does not make the aforementioned offer, you can justifiably call in about an hour after you've left to say that you're still in the waiting room and probably won't make it back in.

Cons: Can't be used too often without arousing suspicion; a nosy boss might inquire about your reasons for seeing the doctor.

Note: A "dentist appointment" is not necessarily interchangeable with a "doctor's appointment." People may expect to hear horror stories or see some sort of physical difference in teeth or gums after an extended trip to the dentist. Furthermore, dentist appointments should not be used in addition to doctor's appointments, but rather as a way of varying your medical reasons for being away from the office.

4 Electrical Outage

Example: "The storm knocked out my electricity while I was sleeping last night, and my alarm didn't go off."

Ideal usage: Buying yourself an extra bit of sleep on a rainy morning.

Duration: Thirty to ninety minutes

Believability: Decent. This has actually happened to just about everyone at some point (or we've all used this excuse at least once, anyway). Either way, your boss can be expected to give you the benefit of the doubt.

Versatility: Can only be used if the weather truly was bad. For those who do not have the good fortune of living in a monsoon zone, it's almost impossible to plan for.

Backstory: Unless you're trying to employ this excuse during perfect weather, there's no need for anything beyond a single sentence.

Frequency: Should be used sparingly, no more than once a year. Overuse will result in your boss thinking that you're either a lazy liar or a complete idiot who can't manage an alarm clock.

Pros: Gives you an excuse for looking bleary eyed and groggy.

Cons: Will only get you a half-day out of the office at best. Not very useful for urban dwellers and others who may live near a coworker who typically arrives on time.

5 **Inclement Weather**

Example: "The roads near my house aren't plowed yet; I'll get in as soon as I can."

Ideal usage: Staying home and making snow angels or curling up in front of a warm TV.

Duration: One to two days.

Believability: So-so. If you're truly snowed in, then you're just telling the truth. If it's questionable, you'd better hope that no one else from your neighborhood made

it to the office that day. If you're in Los Angeles,
you're fired.
Versatility: Being a weather-contingent excuse, this is
not a story you can pull out of the bag at any given
time. Additionally, it's of little use to people in dense
urban settings and of absolutely no use to those in warm
and/or dry climates.
Backstory: The entire excuse hinges on how easily you can
convince your boss of the horrible road conditions so
that there's no need for any elaborate tale-telling.
Frequency: Depending on your local weather conditions and
the efficiency of your local plow drivers, the frequency
varies greatly. For those in remote, wintry regions it
wouldn't be beyond belief to use this excuse twice a
month during the winter season. For those in more temperate
zones, two to three times a season is appropriate.
Pros: It's a perfect way to keep from venturing out into
nasty rain and/or snow. Plus, if the weather's truly bad,
you won't be the only one skipping school.
Cons: One pass of the snowplow or an unexpected appearance
by the sun can ruin your entire plan.

6 **Sick Child/Spouse**
Example: "My wife/husband/child is really ill and I've
got to stay home and keep an eye on him/her."
Ideal usage: As a last resort—when all else fails and you
can't tell your boss the truth.
Duration: One to four days.
Believability: People tend to believe that you wouldn't
lie about your loved ones being ill, so it's easy to take
advantage of their naiveté.

Versatility: Only works for people who actually have spouses and/or children (although a girlfriend/boyfriend could be used in a pinch).
Backstory: This fake illness is obviously a very personal matter, so pleading privacy works just as well as vague statements. ("It's ... well, it's complicated.") However, this is another situation where it couldn't hurt to have a full narrative ready to unfurl. ("Did you know that you can still get leprosy?")
Frequency: Even if you have no qualms about lying about your family's health, this approach is still to be used very rarely—multiple absences will begin to make people either genuinely worried or extremely suspicious.
Pros: Whether it's because they're being kind or they consider you ill by association, your boss may offer you more time off than you're requesting. Additionally, he may see to it that your work is done in your absence.
Cons: You'll more than likely have to deal with well-wishing coworkers when you get back. Also, the person who fills in on your projects may be completely inept, making the workload upon your return all the more onerous.

(7) **Plumber/Landlord**
Example: "My water heater is on the fritz and I've got to be here to let my landlord in to fix it."
Ideal usage: For those days when the mere thought of going to the office makes you ill.
Duration: Four hours to one day.
Believability: Who hasn't wasted an entire day waiting for a plumber or locksmith to show up? No one should doubt your story.

Versatility: Even though the idea is to get out of work for an entire day, this excuse is best for last-minute "I simply cannot do this today" decisions.

Backstory: The chances of anyone wanting to hear about your day spent waiting for a plumber are pretty slim. Even so, it helps to know which bit of plumbing needed fixing in case someone tries to talk shop with you.

Frequency: Another excuse that's more credible the less you employ it. Only to be used very sparingly (once every six months at most).

Pros: Easily allows you to turn "I'll be in at eleven" into "I don't think I'm going to make it in today."

Cons: Since your boss assumes you're at home all day sitting around waiting, don't be surprised to get any number of work-related phone calls. While your boss can most likely relate, it is rarely good to have her picturing you at home watching TV, and you may be expected to work on a project at home while you wait.

Note: If you use this excuse, pray your water heater doesn't break any time in the near future.

Section II

The Longer Lunch:
The Tray of Half-Eaten Food
and Other Time-Wasting Methods

So you've made it to noon and successfully
dodged an entire morning's worth of work.
That's quite an achievement—but remember
that you've got at least five more hours of
time-killing and clock-watching before you can
slip out of the confines of your office and
breathe the sweet freedom of the outdoors.
What's a good Overachieving Underperformer
to do? There are only so many times you can go
home sick or pretend you've got a meeting
away from the office. With that in mind, here
are some methods for adding the right amount
of idleness to those early afternoon hours.

Chapter 7

Lovely Leftovers:
Salvation in a Paper Sack

Generally speaking, it's a given that bosses look more favorably upon employees who work through their lunch hours, scarfing down sandwiches while staring dutifully at their computers. (For some reason, salads make them look even more responsible.) That's precisely why you need to appear to be one of those employees.

One thing you'll learn as you hone your nonworker skill set is to appreciate the value of garbage. Your average person looks at his half-finished lunch or dinner and thinks one of two things, either "I'll wrap this up and save it for tomorrow," or "I'm never going to finish this; might as well toss it." However, the truly wise Overachieving Underperformer will look at said leftovers and think, "You're my ticket to a ninety-minute noontime break tomorrow, and another step toward that big raise when I convince the boss I worked straight through lunch."

1. The next time you don't finish that order of Chinese food, or you make too much pasta for dinner, carefully pack up those leftovers for future use. If you're not going to employ this technique the next day, freeze them. They'll keep even longer and allow you more flexibility—the masterful Overachieving Underperformer will have a full array of frozen leftovers at the ready. (Don't worry about freezer burn; it's not like you're actually going to eat these cast-off scraps.)

2. Bring some frozen delight to the office with you in the morning (preferably in a microwavable container) and leave it out where it will thaw but won't be seen; any one of those empty drawers in your desk will do. When lunchtime finally arrives, wait until your boss and coworkers have begun to leave (make a mental note of who's leaving; this will come in handy), then head for the microwave. Reheat the food until it appears edible and begins to smell; it's a good idea to select very aromatic foods so as to draw attention to yourself. When the food is reheated, take it back to your office and place it in front of your computer, but DON'T SIT DOWN!

3. Getting into character with a slightly distressed look on your face, go around to a few people who haven't left the office yet. Inquire as to the whereabouts of one of the coworkers whom you know is already out to lunch. "Hey, seen Carol around?" When they ask why you're looking for her, just offer up a distracted shrug and walk away in a huff, grumbling, "I can't

even eat my lunch without being distracted ..." Repeat the question to three or four different people and you've planted the idea in their minds that not only are you still in the office at lunchtime, but you're forgoing eating to do work instead.

4. Head back to your desk. Discard (or eat, if you're really hungry) a portion of the leftovers. By now, almost everyone who is going out to eat has left and is in the middle of rushing to chow down and get back to the office. Thus, the chances of your being spotted are minimal, and it's time to make your exit. This would be the perfect opportunity for those with the ability to preschedule e-mail deliveries to employ this technique. When you leave, make sure to sneak out some official-looking papers with you. You'll need them later.

5. If you are able to sneak out and remain undetected, you've got about forty-five minutes of free time before your boss and the rest of your coworkers start getting back to the office, and another twenty before anyone notices that you've been away from your desk. Your absence, of course, is part of the con: Upon your return, pull out the official-looking documents you hid on your person earlier and pretend that you've been off in another part of the office dealing with some "issue" instead of eating your lunch. It might even help to say something to a coworker like, "I've been so busy working on that Thompson thing, my lunch is still sitting on my desk!" You've just bought yourself another thirty

minutes of sitting in front of your computer, surfing the Web, pretending to eat, and getting annoyed at people who come by or call to ask questions. And when your boss catches a lingering whiff of the sorry leftovers you've been enduring while you've been "working through lunch," he'll attribute it all to your unrivaled diligence. He might even insist on ordering a pizza for you too.

Lunch Loafing Essentials

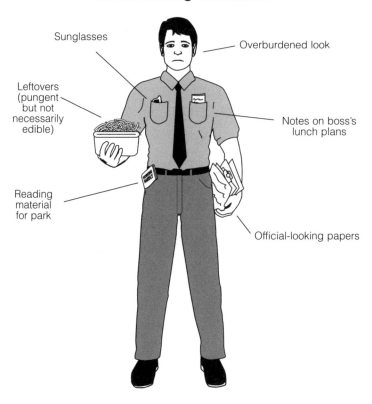

Sunglasses

Overburdened look

Leftovers (pungent but not necessarily edible)

Notes on boss's lunch plans

Reading material for park

Official-looking papers

Chapter 8

Acting 101: How to Look Like You're Working Through Lunch While Writing Your Novel

Most Overachieving Underperformers look for every opportunity to be away from the office, especially at times, like during the lunch hour, when it's not even expected that they'd be at their desk. However, some days you may just not feel like going outside. Maybe it's the weather, or maybe you've just gotten to a really interesting section in that thriller you've been writing. And while most companies don't mind personal use of the computer during lunchtime, why should you waste an ideal opportunity to take advantage of your boss's flawed notion that you're a hard worker?

If you really want to make a misleading impression on your superiors by letting them believe that you're simultaneously eating and working, you'll need to learn a few basic acting tips.

1 Fight Your Instincts

How often have you walked by someone's office and heard her chuckle at something on her computer? Since only a madman (or someone with a much better job than yours) would find working enjoyable, the automatic assumption is that she's reading a personal e-mail, or at least looking at something that is not job-related. While doing so she was unable to fight back the instinct to laugh, thus giving herself away to anyone within ear-shot. This sorry drone has yet to learn the ability to internalize the laughter, to enjoy herself silently, and if she is frequently overheard by her superiors, she may as well forgo any hope of ever getting a raise.

The Overachieving Underperformer, on the other hand, is a master of her emotions—or at least how she displays them. She scowls with equal scorn at a memo from the CFO announcing staff cuts and pictures of her sister's newborn baby. Regardless of what she's pretending to work on, she exudes steely concentra-

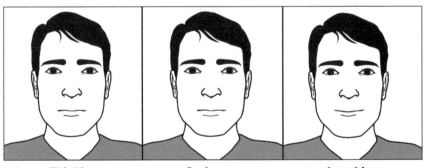

| **Thinking about stumps.** | **Crying on the inside.** | **Laughing hysterically.** |

tion. No one would ever guess that her lunches are spent writing freelance record reviews for some off-beat Web site.

2 The Stare

It's very easy to get sucked into doing something that you enjoy, which is fine until someone interrupts you and you're caught scrambling to hide the screenplay you've been working on all morning. This is why you must develop the ability to appear completely focused on what you're working on while being fully aware of your surroundings. It's an especially important skill if you "work" in a cubicle or shared office.

Honing "the stare" requires that you separate your visual and auditory senses. While your eyes are intently fixed on the monitor, your ears are scanning the vicinity for approaching footsteps or voices. With enough practice you'll begin to recognize the sounds of your boss approaching—the change that always jingles in his pocket; the clomping sound of her shoes drawing nigh—and without hesitation switch to a spreadsheet until the danger has passed.

3 The Toe-Tap

While there are benefits to sitting at your desk during the lunch hour, you might want to get up and stretch a little. But just because you're stepping away from the computer for a few seconds doesn't mean you can't still appear busy.

Say you've finally reached the midpoint of the epic novel you've been saving on your office hard drive. Why not take this chance to print it out? It helps if you print it out in small sections. This way, you'll draw attention to yourself making multiple round trips to the printer, but you won't look as conspicuous as you would carrying all five hundred pages of the saga back to your desk. While you're at the printer, be impatient; keep checking the pages as they spew out. If anyone tries to talk to you, keep your responses as short and to the point as possible. When the printing is done, grab the stack of pages and hurry back to your desk ASAP. If you're in the middle of a conversation, end it abruptly; your pretend work is more important than hearing about someone's high school reunion.

4 Being in the Moment

The best actors are those who not only have their lines memorized and their movements down pat, but also are able to read the other actors and alter their behavior to best fit the scene. The same holds true for the Overachieving Underperformer. Yes, it's important always to look busy when the boss comes strolling by your work space. But what about when she stops to talk to you, not for the purpose of giving you more work, but because she's in a chatty mood and has selected you as the perfect employee with whom to discuss her new sofa?

The danger of becoming ensnared in one of these conversations is highest during the lunch hour, when a boss on her way in or out may be under the misguided impression that you'd *enjoy* taking a break from the hard work you've been doing all morning to exchange vapid blather about some inane thing or other. In such a case, it's to your benefit to put your pseudowork aside briefly and focus on pretending you care what your boss has to say. You needn't actually listen to the words she's forming, only her tone. If she's overly happy, smile and nod your head agreeably—think about a humorous e-mail you recently received. If she's sullen, lean forward in your chair and nod your head thoughtfully—think about the different escape plans you might employ in a few hours to sneak out early. When she's finished her remark, reply, "I agree—that's hilarious!" or "I agree—that's quite sad," as the situation demands. Then sit silently until she moves on.

By spending just one minute pretending to be on your boss's wavelength, you've avoided wasting more time than necessary on her frivolities (rather than your own), while also scoring big personal points with her—points that will prove useful come annual bonus time, or when the boss has to choose someone to represent the department at that convention in Maui. And by silently mulling over your own thoughts while feigning interest in hers, you've killed two birds with one stone.

Planning Carl's Birthday Party:
A Timeline of a Perfectly Wasted Day

An office birthday party is the quintessential time-waster. With a little planning and foresight, you can turn your coworker Carl's birthday into several trips out of the office—and more than three hours away from your desk!

☐ **Tuesday, 3:45 p.m.:** Send out an e-mail to everyone in your department announcing that it's Carl's birthday tomorrow. "Cake 4 Carl's B-Day @ 3:00pm in the conference room!" To seal the deal, add, "Not to worry—I'll take care of everything."

☐ **Wednesday, 11–11:30 a.m.:** Without making an undue fuss about it, let a few of your coworkers know you're stepping out to get the card.

☐ **Noon:** Send another e-mail reminding everyone of the party, and note that you'll be coming around to collect funds and allow your coworkers to sign the card. But make only a brief, halfhearted attempt to collect money so you'll have an excuse to wait until after lunch to complete the job.

☐ **2–2:45 p.m.:** Go to the store to pick up the cake. Before leaving, ask the most irresponsible and absentminded member of the department to pass around the card.

☐ **2:45–3:15 p.m.:** Return to the office and feign frustration that the card is in the same place you left it. Playing the martyr, reluctantly take it upon yourself to get people to sign it. This inevitably delays the beginning of the party, encouraging restlessness in your now-eager coworkers.

☐ **3:15–3:30 p.m.:** Call everyone except Carl into the conference room. Finally, when everyone's ready, ask one of your coworkers (now chomping at the bit to get things started) to fetch Carl for his surprise. Doling out this prominent task serves the dual purposes of fostering the perception that the party was a group effort and suggesting that you're doing this for Carl, not for the glory.

☐ **3:30–4:30 p.m.:** The party begins and coasts on its own energy for about thirty minutes. When the conversation starts to flag, ask Carl, "What time of day were you born?" This is the type of question that will invariably result in everyone offering the specifics of their own births, or explaining why they don't know this information. Such meandering discussions can easily stretch a birthday celebration to over an hour.

☐ **4:30–4:45 p.m.:** As the party nears the breakup point, quietly exit the room and wait a few minutes for people to begin clearing out. At that point, pop your head back in and jokingly remark, "You guys still here?" Stay and volunteer to help clean up. To stretch things out even further, scoop up any palatable remains and offer them around the neighboring departments.

☐ **4:45–5:30 p.m.:** Your entire department is now sluggish and in a bloated, sugar-induced haze. As planned, the party petered out just shy of five o'clock—just past the tipping point beyond which most employees will give up on the day. Coworkers stray from their desks, chatting in the hallway, or prattle away on the phone, discussing anything but office work. Reward yourself with a few games of computer solitaire, then check the birthday database to see how soon you'll have the pleasure of doing it all over again.

Chapter 9

Dine & Dash:
The Culinary Art of Deception

The average worker slogs through his morning waiting for those few brief seconds he'll have to slip away from his desk to eat his lunch. However, to the Overachieving Underperformer the term "lunch hour" is merely a suggestion for the minimum amount of time that should be spent away from the office. There's really nothing to say that one can't have multiple lunch hours on any given day.

1 The Pre-Lunch

Any nutritionist will tell you that breakfast is the most important meal of your day. It's those early-morning nutrients that wake you up and propel you through your daily rigors. But what about those days when breakfast is an impossibility? Or those days when you pretend that breakfast is an impossibility? Well, better late than never.

About an hour before your standard lunchtime, it's time to head to the local market and grab something light to nibble on. Don't make any overt attempts to be seen by your boss or coworkers, but if you are spotted exiting the building, say that you are starving and need a "little something" to get you through the morning. Everyone has been in this situation, and no one will fault you for trying to stay focused and alert in the office.

Bring whatever snacks you've purchased (muffins, fruit, and yogurt are highly recommended for their "sensible" aura) back to your desk and pretend to work while picking away at your food.

- **Time wasted away from office:** ten to fifteen minutes
- **Time wasted at your desk eating:** fifteen to thirty minutes
- **Total time wasted:** twenty-five to forty-five minutes

2 Lunch I

Okay, so now you have food in your stomach. But it was really only a snack, right? It's not as if you ate an entire meal, and if anyone expects you to finish out the day, you're going to need some midday sustenance.

Get to know your coworkers' lunch habits. You'll want to fall in with a small group of people who tend to eat lunch together away from the office. When they congregate before leaving the building at lunchtime, hover in their vicinity until they ask you to come along. This way, even if several members of your Lunch I dining group know that you've already gone out to get something to eat earlier, you'll be seen as a good sport for wanting to be part of the group. More importantly, these same people will unwittingly cover for you when you take another lunch hour later.

- **Time wasted away from office:** forty-five minutes to one hour

③ Lunch II

So now you've returned from the day's second food-related trip outside the office. Common sense would tell you that you've done all you can, and that it's time to find other ways of killing time. Common sense would be very mistaken.

During the fifteen minutes immediately after returning from Lunch I, act extra busy and make sure you're seen hustling and bustling by your boss and any overly nosy coworkers. By the time you've taken care of pretending to be back to work, most of your coworkers will have hunkered down for the afternoon at their desks. Take advantage of the empty hallways and make your exit once more. Again, should you be spotted, claim that lunch has made you sleepy and you need to get some coffee. If anyone points out that you have a coffee machine in your office, sneer and say, "You call that coffee?"

While you're out walking off that deli milkshake or checking out the new releases at the video store, your lunch companions will be back in the office, insisting to your boss that you're around. ("We all came back from lunch at the same time. He must be around here somewhere!")

- **Time wasted away from office:** fifteen to forty-five minutes

 Teatime

Employees who toil away at their desks for three hours after returning from lunch are allowed at least a brief respite to fight off the late-afternoon drowsies. So are Overachieving Underperformers who at this point in the day have already squandered the better part of three hours eating or pretending to do so—provided they followed the OU Code and did so on the sly.

So round about four thirty, take a lap around the office inquiring who might need a little caffeine inspiration. And don't be lazy about it—the more cups of tea or coffee you bring back from your thirty-minute trek to the café, the wider the round of understood applause from grateful coworkers. Be careful to get the requests for cream and sugar correct—these are the people who are going to be covering for your slacking tomorrow.

- Time wasted away from office: thirty minutes
- Time spent distributing tea and coffee: ten to twenty minutes
- Time spent adding sugar to your own cup, reheating it in the office kitchen (must have gotten cold while you were attending to everyone else's beverages), then blowing on the steaming cup as you sit back down at your desk: five minutes
- Total time wasted: forty-five to fifty-five minutes

Chapter 10

The "Interview" and Other Ways
to Get Your Coworkers to Cover for You

Overachieving Underperformers must be able to rely on the kindness of their coworkers. You want them each to think that they share a personal bond with you, that they can depend on you, and vice versa. None of this means you actually have to form these ties with these people, only that you let them believe such ties exist. Why all this talk of pretend brotherhood? Because it means you get to take an extra hour at lunchtime to spend with your real friends.

Suppose for a second that your old college roommate is coming through town for one day only and you've made plans to meet for a catch-up lunch. Now, you're not going to be a doormat and let your employer determine how long said lunch is going to last, are you? Of course not. That means you're going to need someone to cover for you in case you want to have a few extra cups of coffee. Here are a few tactics for ensuring that at least one of your coworkers has your back.

The "Interview"

One of the most secretive and highly sensitive undertakings you can attempt during the workday is to slip out for a job interview at another company. For the Overachieving Underperformer, there are ways to make the transition easier (see next chapter) and excuses that will get you out of the office for a sufficient amount of time (see "Getting Away with It," page 38). But you should never tell a coworker that you're leaving for a job interview. That is, unless you're not actually interviewing.

Select a coworker who counts you as an office friend, but who secretly covets your job. (Be careful not to choose a gossipmonger.) As she'll believe it's in her best interest for you to move out of her way and take a job elsewhere, in your absence this person should be happy to cover for you by saying things like, "Oh, I just saw him at the copier," or, "I asked him to run some documents over to Corporate for me."

Before you head out for your extended lunch, approach her in her work space, shutting the door behind you if possible. Explain to her that you've just gotten called for an interview across town and that you might be back from lunch a little later than usual. If this "friend" doesn't automatically volunteer to cover for you, prod her a little by telling her how you're afraid your boss will notice your absence. This should compel her to assure you that she's got your back; if it doesn't, you picked the wrong person and should really think twice about being her fake friend.

2 The "Personal Matter"

There are fewer things that serve to elevate a semi-friend to the status of bosom buddy than sharing a very personal moment with him or her. When coworkers believe they've suddenly seen a heretofore unrevealed facet of your personality, they are considerably more likely to afford you the same kindness they would an actual dear friend. So why not exploit that generosity?

Again, begin by determining which of your coworkers best fits your needs. For this setup it helps to have someone who is emotional and perhaps a little overly friendly with people in the office. Unlike the coworker in the earlier situation who covers for you out of self-interest, the "personal matter" requires someone who hides your absence because he believes he is doing the proper, friendly thing.

Walk over to his desk to talk to him, and, just as the conversation begins, feign that the cell phone in your pocket is vibrating. Look at the caller ID, bite your lower lip and, sighing, say something like, "Huh ... I'd better take this." Apologizing, answer the phone and begin talking quietly to the nonentity on the other end. Become very concerned and even more hushed in your brief, monosyllabic responses. Out of the corner of your eye, make sure that your coworker is likewise concerned about the distressed behavior you're exhibiting.

After a minute or two end the faux conversation with a terse "Okay ... bye," and hang up the phone.

Linger silently around your coworker's work area, as if formulating your plan of action. (In reality you're just wondering if the restaurant you're going to has salmon on the menu.) And then, as if struck by a sudden epiphany, say something along the lines of, "Look, I've ... well, there's a *personal matter* that I've got to deal with at lunchtime. It might take a little longer than an hour ... I'd tell the boss, but he'd just ask me all these questions I don't want to answer right now." Again, if you've calculated correctly, this should elicit an offer to cover for you when your nebulous noontime activities extend beyond the two-hour mark.

The "Personal Matter"

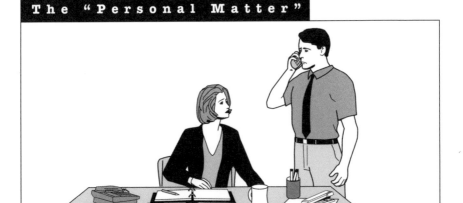

Pretend to get a sudden, unsettling call from a family member.

From Clark Kent to Superman:
Tips for Changing Into Your Interview
Clothes Without Arousing Suspicion

1 **The Professor**

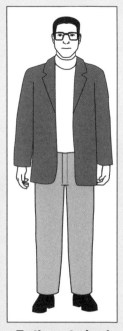

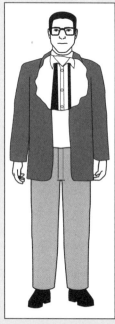

Pros:
- Does not draw attention to wearer
- Can change outfit in less than two minutes
- Easy to change back quickly for return to office

Cons:
- Not good for warm-weather interviews
- Risk of wrinkling shirt and tie
- Bulky and slightly uncomfortable
- Unless you usually wear turtlenecks, can only be used a limited number of times

To the untrained eye this man looks no different (perhaps a little academic) from many other people in the office.

But all he's got to do is ditch the turtleneck and do up his necktie, and he's ready to interview.

The Demure Dresser

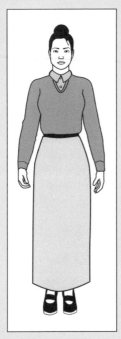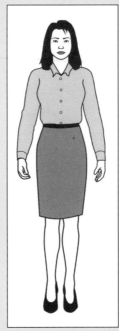

Pros:
- Subtle, inconspicuous
- Virtually no time involved in changing outfits and switching shoes
- Easily restored to original outfit
- Could also be used to conceal slacks

Cons:
- Requires skirt long and capacious enough to conceal interview outfit
- Restricted movement from wearing two skirts
- Must find place to stow outer skirt, sweater, and flats during interview

Sure, it's not terribly eye-catching, but it's also the last thing you'd think she would wear to an interview.

But ten seconds in a phone booth, and she's ready to charm any HR person.

3 The Sloppy/Snappy Dresser

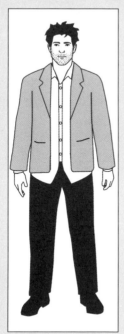

He's well-dressed in that slapdash, youthful way, but there's no way he's going on an interview like that.

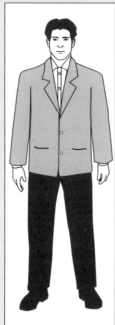

But it's amazing what an electric razor and a comb will do for a man's presentability.

Pros:
- Flexible, good for multiple interviews
- Requires no real change in clothing
- A few days' growth easily shorn in less than five minutes

Cons:
- Only good for end-of-day interviews

Section III
Looking Busy While Doing Nothing

Perhaps you're one of the lucky few who can boast a job that requires little or no work (or better yet, you've got an assistant who can do it all for you). But chances are you're like countless others who have too many tasks and too little time in which to complete them. Regardless of your situation, someone always has more work to give you, and the last thing any sane person would ever want is to have a to-do list loaded up with new items. Myriad strategies exist to combat this conundrum.

Chapter 11

Clutter Is Beautiful:
Simple Steps to a Busy-Looking Office

Most people are operating under the false assumption that maintaining a tidy workplace is essential to looking like a good employee. In reality, an empty in-box is an open invitation for your boss to pile on the work. However, with just a little redecorating, you can convert your office from a space that invites work into one that repels it.

Phase I: Paper = Work

Nothing makes a desk look more foreboding than a mountain range of paper. Some of you may be fortunate enough to have paperwork-intensive jobs where amassing piles of memos and purchase orders is no problem. But in an age in which more and more work is being done without ever having to handle a single page, what's a nonworker to do for clutter? Easy: Make your own!

1. **Downloading clutter:** Print out all your e-mails. Personal or business-related, e-mails look "official" when printed out.

2. **Memos and other company-supplied clutter:** Every corporation drowns its employees in an endless stream of useless memos. Don't take these for granted. Mix them in with your e-mails for added bulk.

CAUTION

As tempting as it may be, never leave anything on your own chair when you're out of the office. This will only draw attention to your absence. If someone actually dares to leave anything on your chair, sit on it long enough to wrinkle the pages, then scold whoever left it there for not putting it in your in-box (which was, of course, overflowing).

---

3 Raiding the recycling bin: For those of you brave enough to get your hands in the paper recycling bin, you've found a treasure trove of clutter to help you on your way!

4 Don't feel confined to busying up just the top of your desk. A truly busy-looking person uses every available surface to his or her advantage.

Using any free chairs in your office is an especially good idea, since it makes it nearly impossible for

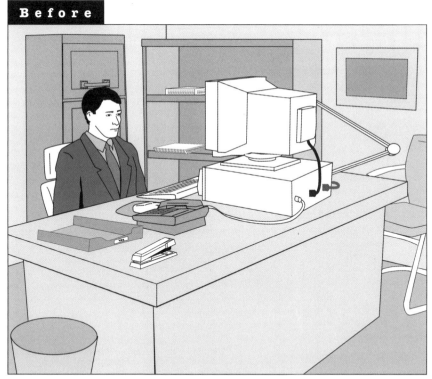

"Fire me; I have nothing but free time."

someone to sit down to "discuss things." As a general rule, you want to make others afraid to visit for fear that some of the work-related clutter might somehow stick to them.

Phase II: The Difference Is in the Details
Your office is looking fantastic, but why not take it to the next level with some fine detail work?

1 **Post-its**
These little bits of sticky paper are a godsend to office nonworkers looking to add some color and realism to their mess. Bright and instantly recognizable, but inconspicuous enough to avoid inspection, Post-it notes can work their magic on just about any surface in your office.

a **Your Computer:** Write down as many names, phone numbers and other reminder memos for yourself as you can, and place the notes around the front edges of your monitor.

 It helps to rotate your Post-it notes randomly every few weeks, just to keep up the illusion that you're working on new projects.

b **Your Shelves and File Cabinets:** Just because your shelves are an unorganized mess doesn't mean your boss needs to know. Create your own cryptic system and label your shelves and file cabinets with Post-it notes for instant credibility. Not only will this artificial organization system help legitimize your mayhem, but also it will discourage snoops and shelf-raiders.

c **Your Desktop Clutter:** Add meaning and importance to those piles of files and papers on your desk. Get a friend to write important-sounding messages on various Post-its, i.e., "Steve, Corporate needs this done ASAP!"

Put these notes on top of the bigger piles on your desk. If someone tries to give you more work, just

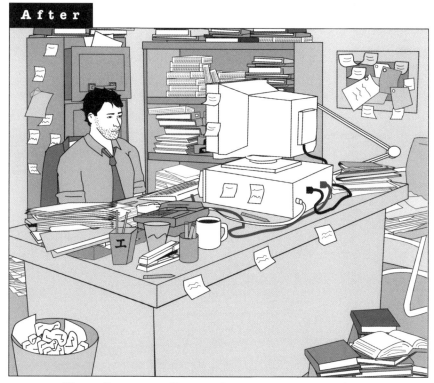

"If you fire me, you'll never find anything in this office."

grunt and point to the now very impressive pile, then tell them that you're busy for the next two weeks.

NOTE: After you attempt the above exercise, you should make a point of gradually decreasing that particular pile over the next few weeks, eventually replacing it with an entirely new stack of "work."

② Virtual Clutter

In the computer age a true Overachieving Underperformer needs to be able to move beyond just making a mess in the physical world. A cluttered desk is vital to looking busy, but it means nothing if you're caught red-handed with a clean, unbusy computer screen.

ⓐ Shuffle up the icons on your computer screen. Only someone with nothing else to do has time to keep all their computer files and folders in order. Since you want to look like someone without an ounce of free time, your computer needs to reflect your faked workload.

ⓑ Create a number of in-progress projects in as many different programs as possible. Having multiple programs and files open at once gives you the appearance of actually having something to do. But more importantly, they also serve as buffers against people who might want to snoop around on your computer while you're out of the office.

Chapter 12

Behind Closed Doors:
Getting People to Leave You Alone

If you're not actually doing most (if any) of the work you're being paid to do, you want to keep snooping eyes as far from your work space as possible. However, there are few things more certain to draw attention to yourself in the workplace than shutting your office door. Secrecy and privacy only breed curiosity and suspicion. That doesn't mean you can't shut your door or keep people out of your office. It just means you have to know what you're doing.

The first step is to let it be publicly known that you're not to be disturbed when you're behind closed doors. You could easily be rude and simply holler at the first person who barges in, but it's better to start off on a gentler setting.

The next time you're on a business phone call, shut the door. Invariably, someone from your office will pick that time to come by and knock. Allow them to open the door a crack (enough to put their head through) and then utilize the classic "on the phone" gesture. Whomever it is will more than likely back off apologetically and wait for you to finish talking. Repeat this several times a day over the course of several weeks, increasing the frequency until every time you're on the phone, the door is closed. Thus, in the minds of those familiar with your work habits, a shut door might as well be a huge neon sign flashing: ON PHONE. COME BACK IN 10 MINUTES. Eventually, most people will stop knocking altogether and just wait until the door is open to bother you. So, whenever you desire a few minutes to take a power nap, scour the Internet for jobs, shop online, read a chapter of your favorite book, or whatever else you can conjure up, it could be just a matter of shutting your door.

Of course, this is not foolproof, as some people are either uneducated or unconcerned about the whole "privacy" issue. These are those intrusive types who knock and enter in one continuous motion, and who continue talking to you even though you're quite obviously in the middle of a phone conversation. It would be easy to simply classify this group as a burden, but it's more productive to view them as an opportunity.

Suppose you've got just about everyone respecting your privacy and leaving you in peace with your newly established shut-door policy. And then, one of these rude knock-and-enterers just barges in on you without warning. You have every right not only to be upset with this person, but also to now lock your door when it's shut. Without question, some of your coworkers will begin to inquire, "Why's your door locked?" Explain that it's necessary to keep those rude party crashers from interfering with your

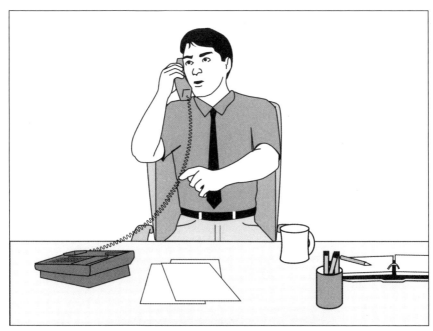

**The classic "I'm on the phone" gesture
is also sign language for "Go away."**

business calls. People will empathize, and they'll begin to follow suit. Soon enough, half of the people in the office will be shutting and locking their doors at every possible opportunity. And if someone's door is shut, it has a tendency to keep that person from leaving his or her office too frequently. This translates into fewer people roaming the halls and more intraoffice phone calls and e-mails, which are considerably easier to ignore.

Overachieving at Underperforming

Some nosy coworkers won't have the decency to stop at merely invading your privacy when you're in your office. This is the particularly crass type of person who, needing something they believe to be in your possession, will walk right into your office *while you're out* and scrounge through your things. All considerations of civility aside, the more pressing concern is that this snoop will uncover some bit of evidence, outing you as a nonworker. A nonworker without a job is not what you want to be.

Having a cluttered mess of an office (see Chapter 11) is a major deterrent to most snoops, but unfortunately not to all. If you're lucky, your file cabinets and drawers have key locks on them. If not, you can employ the "gotcha" tactic: Booby-trapping your office with notes that say things like, "Find what you were looking for?" or, "Would it kill you to ask me if you could rummage through my things?" Hopefully, these will embarrass the nosy nasty into halting her investigation. That being said, a good number of these people haven't even a slight concept of what guilt is. Thus, when she inevitably tells you that she couldn't find that report in your office (because you didn't do it), you should turn the tables on her, changing the topic to the invasion of your privacy and how she's completely messed up your organizational system. If that doesn't work, buy padlocks.

Chapter 13

Identifying and Dealing With
Snooping Coworkers

Wouldn't it be nice if every coworker who intends at some point to rifle through your nonexistent files bore an identifying mark in the middle of his or her forehead? Or if any fusspot who might scour through your computer's hard drive while you're out to lunch was required to declare his or her sneaky nature upon first meeting? Unfortunately, snoops, spies and snitches come in many shapes and sizes. But that doesn't mean that there aren't ways to profile your coworkers and sniff out these dangerous elements.

1 **Gossips**

Common traits: Overly friendly; prone to exaggeration; amiable to all

Snooping technique: More interested in that unopened box sitting on your chair than in whether or not you've been doing your job. Not likely to search through your desk, but might check your Internet browser's history list to see what you've been looking at.

Damage potential: If all you have to hide is that you still haven't written that quarterly report, the Gossip won't care or probably even notice. However, if you're hiding love letters from that cutie in shipping, you're toast.

How to handle: Spend as much time around this person as is bearable. The more you're within earshot, the less likely the Gossip will be to say anything bad about you.

2 **Backstabbers**

Common traits: Congenial but guarded; good listeners; a lean and hungry look

Snooping technique: Will do anything to get the dirt. More than likely the Backstabber's snooping will be done after work hours for maximum privacy.

Damage potential: If the Backstabber unearths sensitive work-shirking secrets or evidence of your out-of-office escapades, he or she can be deadly to a careless Overachieving Underperformer.

How to handle: Lock everything you can in your office. Make sure your computer is password-protected and that the password is *not* your birthday or anniversary. Also, it couldn't hurt to drop hints that you've got this person pegged as a Backstabber;

Backstabbers are less likely to go poring over the papers on your desk if they think you're onto them.

3 Bootlickers

Common traits: Sycophantic; stubborn; subservient

Snooping technique: Will do whatever their superiors ask, simply because it is asked of them. No part of your office is safe.

Damage potential: If the Bootlicker has been sent to your work space on a mission, he or she will execute the mission with uncompromising vigor, leaving no details out in the final report.

How to handle: If possible, try to get the Bootlicker to believe that you are his or her ticket to future success. Failing that, it helps to call this person out for his or her bootlicking ways in a public setting. This will make the Bootlicker much more self-conscious about how others perceive his or her behavior, and thus more likely to curb the more offensive bootlicking tendencies.

4 Micromanagers

Common traits: Nitpicky; egocentric; second-guessers by nature

Snooping technique: Will search through your desk and your computer without permission whenever you're away from your office for more than thirty seconds.

Damage potential: The Micromanager isn't easily fooled by a shiny finished product; he or she may search out evidence of whether or not you actually prepared it. This, obviously, could be disastrous.

How to handle: Install antiquated software on your computer and make it widely known that you prefer using these outdated programs by dropping comments like, "All the bells and whistles on the new applications make my head spin," or, simply, "That's the way I learned, and until I see something better I'm not changing." Then fill a file or two with garbled text and save them using a naming convention that would associate the files with your current projects. The benefits here are several: Anyone who comes snooping will find the files but be unable to make any sense of them. You've also got a ready excuse for why it always appears that someone else has prepared your work—you had to have an assistant/colleague convert it into a file that the rest of the office could use. And your devotion to old-fashioned programs might even earn you bonus points for "eccentricity"!

5 **Assistants: aka Innocent Assassins**

Common traits: Naïve; unquestioning; gullible

Snooping technique: Obliviously going through your files under the assumption that anyone is allowed to sift through your stuff.

Damage potential: While these well-meaning folks couldn't hurt you if they tried, Assistants have a tendency to unearth that one damning file that could unhinge years of carefully constructed deception.

How to handle: Preemptive strike: Whenever a new assistant is hired, immediately make it clear who has permission to be in your office (no one) and which items are cleared for general perusal (none).

Chapter 14

The "Big Project": Exploiting Massive Corporate Bureaucracies for Your Benefit

In between the pampered executives and the lowliest peons, most large companies are overloaded with people all doing variations of the same job. Most of these caught-in-the-middle employees are part of a mammoth paper-pushing machine that simply moves files and forms laterally from department to department. (Inventory places orders through Production, which talks to Purchasing, which deals with Operations, etc.) Thus, once you land such a position, most of the people who are bringing you work to do are at or around your same general rank and responsibility level. Why is this not a negative? Simple. Because of all the redundancies in staffing, if you're overloaded with work, it's quite easy to convince others to bypass you and pass the work on to one of your peers. Of course, as you've seen, one need not actually *be* overworked for people to think you are overworked.

1 The "Big Project"

Whether it's at the end of the fiscal year, before a seasonal product launch, or during an annual inventory audit, every company experiences brief periods of intense workloads during which everyone's focus shifts from daily tasks to special assignments. With so many employees being forced to handle new and unusual chores, people can lose track of exactly who is doing what and for whom. Additionally, since most corporate employees find themselves being pushed around by several supervisors (see Chapter 15), each with his or her own agenda, the Overachieving Underperformer can take advantage of this to pull off the ironic charade of the "big project"—using the fact that everyone has so much work on their plate to avoid tasting even a morsel of it yourself.

Suppose it's the end of your company's fiscal year. Someone comes to you with expenditure reports that need reviewing. Tell them you're already saddled with, for example, a productivity-analysis file to check. Regardless of what people try to dump onto your lap, there's always some other facet of the "big project" that you can talk up to sound more urgent and pressing than whatever is in their hands. And because these people are fretting and haven't got the time to check the veracity of your claims, you can make it through to the other side of this particular maelstrom without so much as a paper cut.

2 The "Backlog"

The one characteristic of paperwork is that it always has to be passed on. That form must be signed by twenty different people in four different offices in order to be of any use. (That's if it was of any use to begin with.) However, that doesn't mean you can't make photocopies of said forms and keep them on your desk for those afternoons when you really need some "me" time. Should anyone come to you attempting to foist more work on your shoulders, merely flash the photocopies, and comment, "These all came back from Distribution unsigned, but no one will tell me why. It's gonna take all afternoon to sort through it and figure out what went wrong." Even if that person refuses to give your work to someone else, you've at least got a good excuse for not touching it until the next morning.

3 The "Policy Change"

If there's one thing for which massive corporations can be relied upon, it's inane policy changes with little or no notice for those involved. Thus, when Sadie from Inventory comes to your office bearing a load of paperwork that would kill a mule, try telling her that you're no longer supposed to receive those particular forms without the new routing slip. She'll of course claim that she hasn't heard anything about it (because you just made it up). To this, merely shrug your shoulders and say, "Rules are rules." She'll go back upstairs, cartload of papers in tow. By the time she figures out that you were not telling the truth (claim that it was a nasty rumor, of which you were both innocent victims), it will be too late in the day for you to even think about looking at all the work. Hopefully it's something that's needed in a rush (or that you can *pretend* is needed in a rush) and you can enlist the help of your coworkers (read: get them to do it for you).

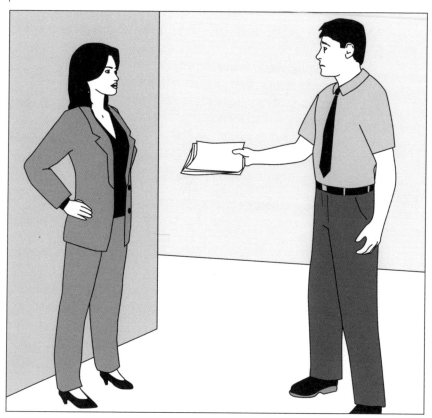

Refuse to accept any work that doesn't come with a routing slip. By the time your coworker realizes there's no such policy, you'll be at the bar.

Tetris, Minesweeper, and Solitaire (aka The Trinity)

Sure, there are countless games available for your computer. Yet somehow, everyone has at some point found themselves caught up in a Minesweeper marathon, declared, "This is my last game of solitaire, and then back to work ... I swear," or been entranced for hours on end by the falling colored Tetris blocks. Why are these games so universal? Simple: Because they're free and they come preloaded onto just about any PC you buy.

 Tetris

The basics: Multicolored orthogonal shapes descend one at a time from the top of the screen to the bottom. The player rotates these pieces and moves them horizontally to get them to interlock. The speed of the blocks' descent increases as the game progresses.

Pros:

- You control the game using the arrow keys on your keyboard; less noticeable than a mouse click.
- With any amount of practice, the average Tetris game takes at least five minutes of your workday and will continue until you can no longer keep up with the computer.
- Relatively lengthy games are easy to get sucked into—good for taking your mind off all the work you're not doing.

Cons:

- Has a tendency, especially at advanced levels, to get players too excited, especially after one breaks a previous high score or angrily loses a twenty-minute Tetris session.

- While you can easily alt-tab to another application if someone unexpectedly interrupts you, the game will continue playing unless you pause it first.
- The rapidly moving pieces and bright colors look nothing like a spreadsheet and are immediately noticeable.

Tips:
- Pause the game between every level and look away from the monitor for a few seconds. This will extend the length of the game and help prevent the glassed-over stare that comes with playing too much Tetris.
- Even though the game only requires one hand on the keyboard, remember to keep your other hand in position near the keyboard so that your body language does not give you away.
- Make sure that you turn off any associated sound effects or mute the sound entirely on your computer; one loud "bloop" could mean your job.

2 **Minesweeper**

The basics: A predetermined quantity of "mines" (ten for beginners, fifty for medium, ninety-nine for advanced) are hidden within an array of gray squares. By clicking on these squares and following the numerical clues that are uncovered, a player marks the mines and clears all the safe squares.

Pros:
- Even the large, advanced-level screen only occupies a small portion of your monitor, and the subtle gray tones will not draw unwanted attention.
- Game play goes quickly, often lasting less than a few minutes; there's no extensive time investment required if you're only after a quick fix.

- Requires a modicum of brain power to win; passersby may think you're actually concentrating on the work you've given someone else to do.

Cons:

- Tends to encourage repeated playing; you may find that you've spent an entire day playing Minesweeper and missed several online auctions for record albums you want.
- The endless mouse clicks are a dead giveaway. Anyone who's informed and listening knows you're playing Minesweeper.
- The advanced level tends to frustrate players to the point of visible agitation. Don't get fired because you couldn't locate all ninety-nine mines.

Tips:

- Don't try to beat the clock. If you can keep your play at a moderate pace, the mouse clicks are less noticeable.
- Don't be greedy. Once you break one of your previous records, stop playing for at least a few minutes. Don't you have a personal phone call to make?
- Stick to playing the medium and advanced levels as much as possible. The beginner's level is too easy and fosters speedy clicking.

3 Solitaire

The basics: Solitaire includes any number of one-player card games that involve sorting a randomly shuffled deck into numerical order by suit.

Pros:

- No time clock and no moving pieces, so you can play at your own pace. No need to pause before you alt-tab.
- Most PCs are packaged with an array of solitaire games; variety is the spice of clock-watching.

- Can usually be played with either the mouse or the arrow keys.

Cons:
- There's not a boss on this planet who doesn't instantly recognize the solitaire screen. Be seen playing and you *will* get busted.
- Because most solitaire hands are not winnable, most people will continue to play until they win at least once. You might find yourself playing hand after hand of solitaire instead of taking a much-needed snack break or making idle chitchat with your coworkers.
- Players have a tendency to forget what they're doing and concentrate on the game instead of looking busy.

Tips:
- Never take your left hand off the alt-tab key combination. You might want to occasionally interrupt your game with a quick jump to another open program just for practice.
- Learn to play the game with a combination of keystrokes and mouse clicks. This will help prevent giveaway body language (solitaire "tells") and will sound like you're just doing normal work.
- Take your time; it's less obvious and you may learn some good strategies if you stop and think about your next move.

Chapter 15

Billy Has Two Bosses:
Playing Your Superiors Against Each Other

For many corporate employees, having only one supervisor is an aberration. You probably have two or more bosses nagging you daily, and perhaps another higher-level micromanager above them who feels compelled to periodically check on your productivity. The average worker would complain and say that this disparate control only causes confusion. The Overachieving Underperformer would agree with that argument but would definitely not complain about it. Here is a little story to illustrate:

Billy has two bosses.

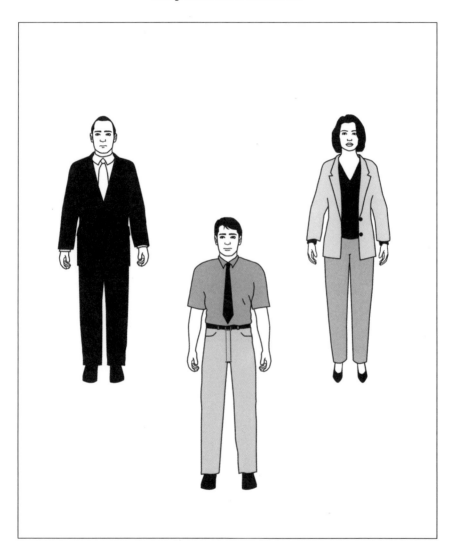

Billy's bosses don't get along.

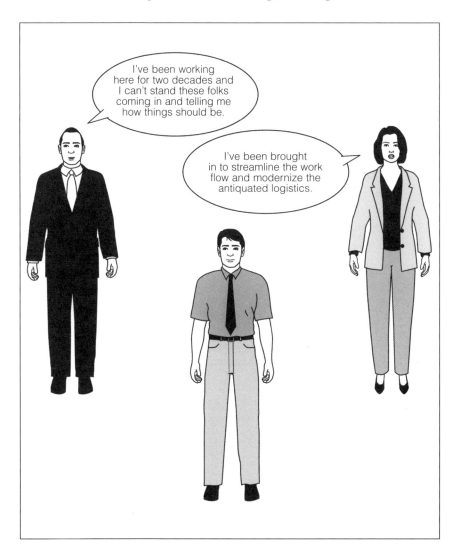

**Billy knows just the things to say
to make sure they never get along.**

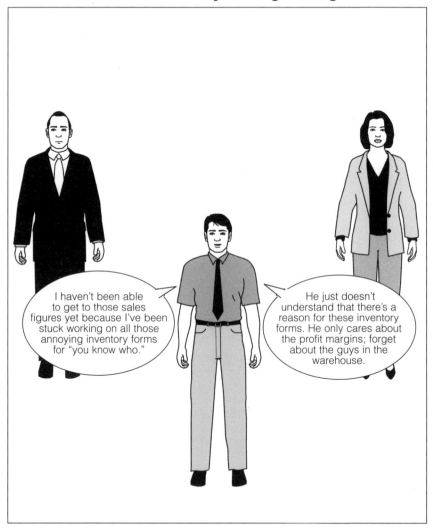

Looking Busy While Doing Nothing

Billy isn't going to do any work today, and probably none tomorrow.

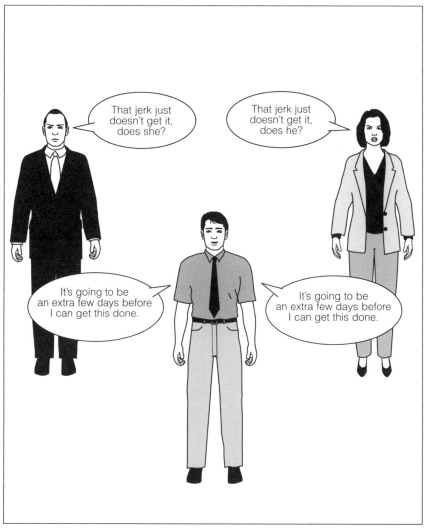

Chapter 16

Exploiting the "Home Office" and Other Corporate Bogeymen to Get Others to Do Your Work

Fear of the unknown is a great motivator, as is the fear of losing one's job. For the Overachieving Underperformer who can successfully combine and exploit these two fears within the setting of a large, multinational corporation, the reward is never having to do a tedious report or spreadsheet ever again.

Let's say your boss has asked you to sift through a pile of data and summarize the information in a memo. You do not want to do this. Solution? Find someone else. Consider these basic truths:

Fact #1: As an employee of a mammoth conglomerate, more than likely you're working in a branch office that reports to a regional managing office, which in turn reports up the totem pole to some mysterious entity of which people speak in hushed tones, known generically as the "Home Office" or "Corporate."

Fact #2: This highest level of the company food chain often operates mysteriously, only occasionally deigning to dump some cumbersome task on the regional offices. The power that these executives possess to summarily fire staff, or to shutter an entire branch, engenders fear and anxiety in the employees.

Fact #3: Immediately after a decree comes down from above, people have a tendency to fall into line, working more quickly and with increased focus. And, lucky for you, they also tend not to ask too many questions.

Manipulating this scenario is simple. Begin by selecting your target. You're going to need someone who is the person you pretend to be: eager, intense, detail-oriented. Entry-level employees fresh out of college (who probably

---

WARNING
When it comes to pushing off work, avoid anyone who even slightly registers on your OU Meter. Like you, these people will gladly offer to help and then spend two weeks dodging your phone calls.

---

know your job better than you do) and new hires (who often crave something to do so they feel they fit in) are a good place to start.

Next, exaggerate. Play up the importance of whatever it is you're trying to unload on your coworker(s). Make them believe that this is part of a picture so huge that no one really knows what it's all about, and that there's just no way you could possibly handle it all on your own.

Make it known repeatedly that this is an Official Decree from the Powers That Be at Corporate HQ. If you're feeling particularly bold, you might add that this undertaking could decide the fate of your department, or even your entire office.

TIP *If you know the name of some menacing Director of Operations or VP of Finance—one of those people whom everyone has heard of, but few have proof actually exists—use that person's name as if he's the devil incarnate. If you don't know the name of such a person, make one up; if you're convincing, no one will fact-check you.*

Finally, ensure the code of secrecy. Secrets build bonds between the people who hold them. They also make whatever lie you've told that much harder to uncover.

Analysis: Your work is now getting done faster and at a higher level of quality than before. Even better, it's getting done this way by someone else and you're getting all the credit. Now you've got the free time to plan your trip to Italy, which you can afford when that raise comes through.

Chapter 17

Grassroots Complaining:
The Tactical Distribution of Bitching and Moaning

To be a fully functional Overachieving Underperformer requires an insurrectionist's zeal. You must always keep in the front of your mind that you are locked into an Us vs. Them struggle; with the notable exception of paying you to sit at a desk, there is nothing your employer does that is beyond reproach. Thus, it is your duty to be ever mindful of the ways in which your superiors exploit employees. From devastating benefits cuts to minor alterations in office procedure, there is no such thing as a day without something worthy of complaining about.

However, it should be noted that while being an Overachieving Underperformer requires a revolutionary mindset, it also requires that you let others handle the actual revolt. You hate your job, but you can't very well afford to lose it. Thankfully there's an easy-to-follow process for stoking the flames of mutiny without being tried for treason.

(1) **Spin Cycle**

As has been discussed, if you have a day at work when there's nothing to gripe about, either you're not looking hard enough or you're in the middle of a dream and should wake up, because the boss is about to tap you on the shoulder. Look around your office:

- Is there not enough light? Too much light?
- What about the room temperature? It's a little stuffy, right? Or perhaps there's a draft?
- Are the supervisors making too much noise? Or are they disturbingly silent?
- Does your boss micromanage every minute detail of your job? Or is she too hands-off?
- Is your boss aloof and distant? Or is she too familiar and overly friendly?
- Are men and women treated fairly by the company's policies? Maybe one gender is getting an unearned leg up?

Obviously there are no right or wrong answers to any of these questions (and there are countless others begging to be asked); rather, it's a matter of determining which answer you can spin into a bigger, more motivating issue. For instance, suppose you're not getting enough natural light in your area of the office. More than likely it's because all the offices with decent exposures are occupied by higher-ups, and the rank and file is left to toil under the pallid, sickly glare of fluorescent lighting.

So, take your lack of natural light and consider how to expand upon it, how to get your coworkers upset about the blatant injustice: "They don't want us to see the sun because they want us to just sit in our cubicles and work nonstop."

Or perhaps you hunger for the steady luminescence of a carefully calibrated lamp fixture: "How in the world do they expect us to get any work done with the sun pouring through the window like that? I can't even see my monitor because of the glare!"

Either of these statements will start some of your coworkers on a downward spiral of antiestablishment

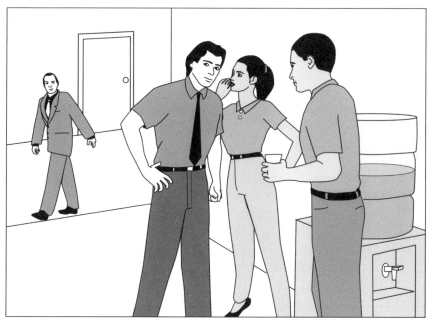

Secrecy and suspicion are the keys to stoking the flames of office insurrection.

anger. This is the desired effect. However, since it would mean putting your paycheck in peril to be seen as an instigator, it's best to have someone else do the most vocal complaining for you.

2 The Patsy

You know that coworker of yours who seems to be constantly starving for a reason to fly off the handle? The one with the hair-trigger temper who sneers at the mere mention of your boss's name? Every office has at least one of these people, if not several, and these are the folks you want to approach first. With someone like this, it's probably not even necessary to over-spin your complaint. Chances are they'll be out the door and griping to others within a matter of seconds, adding their own exaggerations for inflammatory effect. Depending on the size of your office and the audacity of the trumped-up charge, within a day everyone will have heard about it, and a few others will have picked up the banner of your cause.

Occasionally these hot-tempered types are either terribly unlikable or terribly introverted, meaning that either no one listens to their complaints or no one is even told. In such unfortunate cases, you've got some legwork to do. Move to the next desired category of coworker: office gossips. These are people who are generally congenial and well-liked, if only because no one wants to miss out on any of their dirt. That being said, you'll still want to cover your butt. Regardless of whom you choose to start your complaining with, you never want to be known as the source of the complaint. Thus you'll want to start every conversation with a blame-deflecting statement along the lines of, "I was just talking with Charlie. He's awfully bent out of shape about how dark it is in his cubicle ... I dunno; maybe he's right." This way it appears that you are casually reporting something you've observed about the behavior of a third party, and not actually leading the mutinous charge.

3 Picking up Steam

If your grassroots complaint campaign is successful (and it may take several rounds of compiling complaints before the results become evident), there will be a visible downturn in productivity as a palpable anger toward the supervisors coalesces.

Whatever the burning issue may be, it can—when well stoked—grow from an ember into a bonfire. Normal workaday matters such as arriving on time or even doing your job may become secondary to special meetings between management and labor or Q&A sessions to address employees' concerns. All the while, you're taking full advantage of the disruption in productivity to make long-distance phone calls and use the company's courier account to send parcels to relatives in remote parts of the world.

4 Who? Me?

Keep a close eye on the mood of the office. As soon as you realize that the professional proletariat has enough momentum to move forward on its own, fade into the background. Stay in your office and keep to yourself. Thus, when your boss begins to notice your coworkers lingering amid whispers for drawn-out periods of time at the coffee pot and then instantly falling silent and dispersing when he approaches, he might very well turn to you in an attempt to understand why. If this happens, explain to him that you've heard talk of people being upset about something or other, but stress that you're not exactly sure what that something or other is. At the very least, you've given your boss the idea that you're a solid employee who is not swayed by rabble-rousers.

Ideally you'll be asked to take time from your hectic schedule ("But with everyone so distracted, I've had to take on some of their work too!") to speak to your irate coworkers. Should that happen, you'll need to be prepared to argue the complete opposite of your original complaint. There's a chance they might view you as a turncoat or a coward; but sly Overachieving Underperformers would turn this to their advantage, starting the process all over again, complaining about how they were coerced by management into taking sides against their coworkers ("They threatened to take away my 401k!"). Eventually you'll be forgiven (if not martyred) by your colleagues and will have enjoyed a workless week watching this office soap opera unfold. And if your intervention at the crisis's peak managed to quell the unrest, you might even be promoted to a higher-paying nonjob.

Chapter 18

Quid Pro Quo:
Identifying Other Overachieving Underperformers and Methods of Mutual Back Scratching

The life of an Overachieving Underperformer can at times be a solitary existence. But as much as it may seem that it's you against the hardworking masses, you should always keep the following in mind: You're not alone. Unless you're working in a very small office, there are always a couple of like-minded folks, people who understand that having a reputation as a hard worker is just as good (if not better) than actually being one. And while all Overachieving Underperformers ultimately need to look out for number one, there are several benefits to having other idlers in your midst. However, before you start sharing your shirking, you should take a minute to learn some tips on identification.

Jimmy vs. Sally:
Who's the Overachieving Underperformer?

Jimmy

- Comes into the office about thirty minutes late every morning but stays a little later at the end of the day to make up for it.
- Is always openly griping about your boss, paperwork, and anything else that peeves him.
- Has been in the same position for five years.
- Seems to spend a good deal of his time away from his desk, talking socially with other coworkers.
- Is always forwarding you funny e-mails and links to bizarre Web sites.

Sally

- Always in the office by the time you arrive in the morning. Usually leaves promptly at five fifteen, but occasionally stays late to finish her work.
- Makes clever, sarcastic comments about her working conditions, but never seems to be too bothered by all the minor irritations.
- Has been promoted twice in three years.
- Appears to be constantly in the middle of something; only occasionally bothers to make idle chitchat with people in the office.
- Is always the one to take charge of office birthday/retirement/anniversary parties.

To the untrained eye, Jimmy would appear to be a good partner in crime. However, if you've been paying attention, it should be quite obvious that Sally is the Overachieving Underperformer in your office and Jimmy is just a slacker (and one who probably does as much, if not more, work than Sally, but gets a fraction of the credit). And where Jimmy puts no effort into concealing his disdain and sloth, Sally understands the value of putting a happy face on a bad situation. Which one would you rather have as an ally?

Now the question is: What good can you and Sally do for each other? Consider the following scenarios:

1. **Extended Hours**

   Fact: Sally's an Early Bird (see Chapter 5), you're a Late Stayer (see Chapter 20).

   Desired outcome: You both want people to think you're working more hours than you actually are.

   Method: Easy. Sally covers for you in the a.m., ensuring that your lights and computer are on, and stalling your superiors if a crisis arises that demands your presence. When asked by someone else if she's seen you, she noncommittally replies, "Oh yeah ... I think so; over by Accounting." You cover for her in the p.m., checking to make sure her in-box doesn't fill up because she lit out thirty minutes earlier than usual. If Sally has e-mails ready to be sent, you can wait until you're leaving and simply click on "Send All" for her.

   Final result: If all goes according to plan, both you and Sally will appear to be working very long hours. At the very least this will bolster your reputations as dedicated employees. At best you'll both see an increase in pay, perhaps even promotions.

2 Shared Glory

Fact: You've just had someone else write a huge profitability report for you and the boss is thrilled with your work.

Desired outcome: In addition to looking like a corporate superstar, you want to be seen as a team player. But you see that there is no benefit in giving credit to the person who actually did the work.

Method: When being thanked for your efforts on the report, proudly tell your boss that you appreciate the gratitude, but that you "couldn't have done it without Sally's help." If asked what part Sally played in producing the report, be very vague, using terms like "invaluable background research" and "multilayered data analysis"—chances are your boss's eyes will glaze over and he or she won't ask any more questions.

Final result: Not only have you received undue credit for solid work, but also you've portrayed yourself as a humble and gracious believer in teamwork. Sally will also be seen in the same light, especially since she didn't crassly step forward and lay any claim to her nonexistent work. Meanwhile the person who actually performed the task for you (and who thinks he was only working on a portion of a larger project) will simply assume that Sally must have been saddled with an even more critical part of the report. With any luck this coworker will want to be like Sally and will humbly volunteer to assist you in a greater capacity on future items.

The Job Reference

Fact: You're interviewing for a new job and need a reference from your current employer. Thus you'll need Sally to lie for you. Sally wants your current job (because it requires even less work than hers and pays more). Thus, she'll tell someone you invented electricity if it will help her.

Desired outcome: You get a job offer so you can either change companies or use it as leverage to get a raise or a promotion from your current employer.

Method: On your resume, list Sally under a different name with a more important job title. So long as she sounds like a convincing boss, there'll be no need to doubt her. When she is contacted by a potential employer, she'll make it clear that you are a talented and gifted employee whose talents and gifts are sadly going to waste because of the lack of opportunity in your current situation. She will tell them how upset she and the other executives would be to lose such a go-getter, but that she'd understand if you had to move on for the betterment of your career.

Final result: Sally's telephonic acting is so convincing that you are offered this new job. If you really want to change employers, you make the switch and Sally takes over your position. If you're just using the job offer to get more money from your current company, you can return the favor to Sally by referring her to this other company and doing everything you can to make sure she gets the job.

Chapter 19

Hide-and-Go-Sleep:
Securing Nap Zones Within the Office

As office taboos go, sleeping on the job holds a position only barely below embezzlement. To be caught mid-nap during work hours is definitely sufficient grounds for firing; it's irresponsible and it's selfish. This is precisely why you need to be careful about where you nod off.

TIP *The most vital tool for safely locking down nap zones is either a cell phone with an alarm function or a battery-powered alarm clock.*

1   The Toilet

Depending on the cleanliness of your particular office, and how badly your body cries out for a few minutes of shut-eye, the toilet may be the perfect place for that midday snooze.

When you decide to take a toilet nap, leave your desk with—as always—important-looking papers in hand. If you have several lavatories from which to choose in your office, select the one farthest from your desk. This will reduce the odds of others recognizing your shoes under the stall doors.

Position yourself comfortably on the seat. Leaning forward with your elbows resting on your knees is recommended. If you fall into too deep a sleep, your arms will most

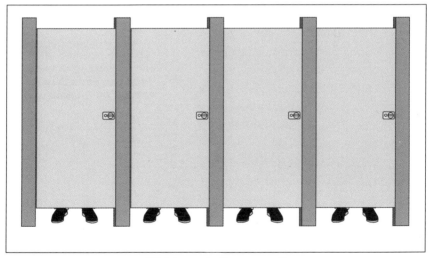

Which one's the napper?

likely slip off to the side, jolting you awake before you fall to the floor.

 The Empty Office

There's a tendency for office workers to be jealous of their bosses' spacious offices: the windows, the big desk, the chair that doesn't require daily doses of back medicine, and quite possibly a couch. There's also usually quite a bit of envy regarding

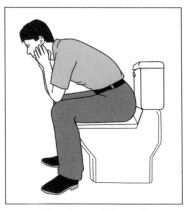

Prior to nodding off, lean forward with head in hands and elbows resting on the knees.

how often the boss is out of the office, whether it be on vacation or some "business" errand. However, whereas the average worker is too busy to see beyond the wasted office space and excessive luxury, the Overachieving Underperformer sees a solid forty winks.

This is a situation where it helps to be overly familiar not just with your boss, but also with executives in other departments. Here is an example of how to use small talk to squeeze the desired information from the VP of Sales:

OU: "I was reading this article on Hawaii the other day ..."
Boss: "I'm sorry ... did you say something?"
OU: "Just saying that I'd really like to go to Hawaii some day. Ever been?"
Boss: "Yeah, about five years ago."
OU: "Lucky you! Any plans for this year?"
Boss: "Going to Greece for a week in May."
OU: "Wow ... That just sounds fantastic ..."

In a few short seconds you've discovered that she will be going away for a week and that she'll be out of the country (and thus less likely to make an early return), and you have a general time frame of when she'll be gone. When May draws near, it only requires a couple more lines:

OU: "Heard it's beautiful in Athens this time of year."
Boss: "I'm sorry ... did you say something?"
OU: "Just saying that I heard Athens is really pretty in the spring."
Boss: "It had better be. I'll be there next Tuesday."

And there you have it, the precise timing for when her office will be vacant and ready for you to collapse behind its shut door, dreaming of how nice it is in Athens.

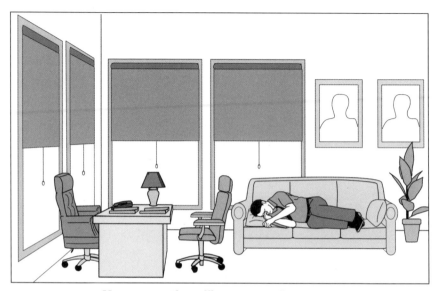

Many executive offices are outfitted with comfortable couches. The key is knowing which executive is out of town.

③ Picking Up the Pieces

Sure, you can go hunting for a free toilet stall, or you can stake a claim to the couches of out-of-town executives. But what about those times when you need to sleep ASAP, and the toilet just isn't going to suffice?

WARNING: This method requires an office with a door that opens inward. Those in cubicles or with outward opening doors will only look silly.

Lie down on the floor of your office with the bottom of your feet touching the door. Get into a comfortable position, one in which a nap should not be too difficult. Scatter some sort of office supplies around your head. Paper clips and rubber bands are best. Tacks and staples, while not unusable, provide a much higher potential for physical injury.

And now take your nap. With any luck, you'll arise forty-five minutes later feeling refreshed and having wasted a decent chunk of your day. However, should anyone attempt to enter your office while you're asleep, your feet up against the door will serve the dual purpose of blocking entry and waking you up instantly. When this happens, snatch up a handful of paper clips and inch forward so that the door opens wide enough for your visitor to pop her head in. When she asks what you're doing, point out to her the scattered paper clips and say, "Picking up this stuff I dropped."

NOTE: If the attempts to open the door do not roust you from your slumber immediately, drastic action is called for. As you finally come to, do not attempt to stand. Instead, act groggy and confused, and claim that you've no idea how you ended up on the floor. The scattered office supplies will add to the general confusion and thus heighten the believability of your story. Mumble that you forgot to eat lunch and perhaps your blood sugar is low. Whatever the excuse, you should be able to translate this potential embarrassment into a trip home to rest for the remainder of the day.

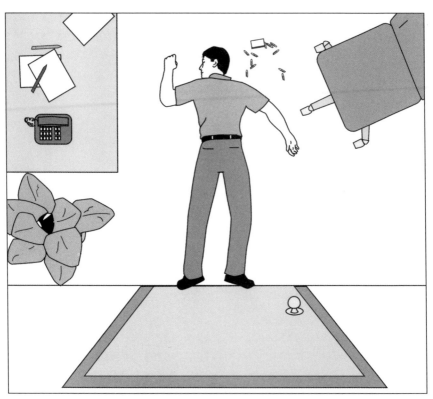

**The "Picking Up the Pieces" technique offers a sound sleep
with a built-in fail-safe to avoid discovery.**

Chapter 20

Burning the Midnight Oil:
The Late Stayer

One of the primary goals in an Overachieving Underperformer's day is to spend as much time away from his or her desk and as little time in the office as possible. However, as discussed earlier, there are significant gains to be made by coming in early or "working" through your lunch hour. Thus, when it comes to working late, widely held preconceptions about what it is to be a "hard worker" are to be used to your advantage.

Just as the Early Bird arrives before his coworker and thus gets to leave before everyone else, the Late Stayer gets to crawl in later in the morning because he was "here so late last night." And where the Early Bird earns points by being ostensibly responsible and dedicated, the appeal of the Late Stayer is that willingness to go the extra mile, forgoing evening plans for the good of the company. So while you might just be killing time until that seven thirty movie or you're waiting for your inlaws to catch their nine o'clock flight back home, everyone in your office will be impressed with your hardiness.

The Early Dinner

So you're going to pretend to work late? That means you'll need sustenance before digging in for the evening. About forty minutes before the end of the day (for everyone else but you), put on your coat and pay a few visits around the office. When your coworkers inevitably ask where you're going so early, make it clear to them that you're only running out to grab some food for your all-nighter.

You've now been given a solid excuse for being out of the office for twenty to thirty minutes. When you return, but before you sit back down at your desk, make certain to be seen still in your coat and carrying your dinner.

NOTE: Try not to speak to the same coworkers before and after getting food. It's generally a good idea to spread out your conspicuousness, and it will not appear as if you're trying to remind everyone what a nose-to-grind-stone employee you are.

Once you've gotten your dinner back to your desk, it should be just about time for everyone else to begin the trek home. Hopefully your work space is in a high-traffic area so as to maximize the number of curious coworkers stopping to ask what you're doing. And just by having your dinner a little earlier than normal, you've not only managed to put it into your coworkers' heads that you'll be working while they sleep, but also you've wasted the last hour of your day with impunity.

In an ideal situation your entire office staff goes home within the same forty-five minute span. In this case all you've got to do is wait out that last coworker and, as soon as she's hit the road, you're free to go. No one will have any reason to doubt that you stuck around for five more hours. Unfortunately it doesn't always work that way, and you might end up actually having to be in the office later than planned because your dinner reservations aren't until eight o'clock. But don't think for a second that you'll be required to do any work.

2   Whiling Away the Hours

Should you find yourself in the position where you physically need to remain at work (whether because you're waiting around for later plans or in order to earn your Late Stayer stripes), there are a number of ways to pass the time. Aside from the obvious tasks of writing personal e-mails and scouring the Internet (this time without the fear of anyone looking over your shoulder), you can commandeer the phone system and make all the personal, long-distance, and international calls you desire.

Overachieving at Underperforming

If you're going to abuse the phone system after hours, it will be to your advantage to use phones in your coworkers' now vacant offices, being sure to distribute the calling over as many extensions as possible.

If there's a nighttime cleaning staff in your office, take this time to familiarize yourself with them on a personal level. After all, who else can get you into your boss's office after hours to slip that overdue report (that you had someone else write) under his blotter? And when, after catching a movie and drinks with your friends, you stop by the office at ten thirty p.m. to compose a "look how late I worked" e-mail, who's going to let you in even though you don't have a key to the building?

Just like anything worth pretending to do, earning a reputation as a Late Stayer can take time. However, once your coworkers finally have you categorized as such, it's not so easy to change their minds. So long as you continue to be one of the last out at the end of the day, you'll be looked upon favorably as a can-do, go-to employee whose first priority is work, when in actuality you're an oversleeper who doesn't mind lingering in the office for a few extra minutes.

Tricks of the Trade

The Shut Door
and Tape Recorder

For the truly brave Overachieving Underperformer: Once you've gotten your coworkers used to leaving you alone when the door is closed, you might want to attempt a bit of audio trickery. Using either a tape recorder or voice-recording software on your computer, make several recordings of yourself reading from the business section of the newspaper. Change your voice slightly, or if you're very tech-savvy, alter it digitally so it almost sounds like you, but not quite. The next time you feel the need to skip out of the office for a few minutes, play this recording at a low volume with your door shut. Someone walking by will assume it's you talking on the phone. But if someone dares to violate the sanctity of your empty office, your coworker will think it's just a news broadcaster who sounds a bit like you.

Section IV
It's Nice to Be the Boss:
Using Your Assistant
to Do Even Less

Up to this point, we've stressed the importance of knowing the appropriate times in which to be conspicuous (i.e., when it's to your advantage to be noticed by your boss) and, conversely, those times when your needs are best served by flying under your supervisor's radar. And while the basic idea behind all of this deception is to allow you to maintain your paycheck while minimizing the actual work you do, the ultimate goal for those willing to shirk the hardest is promotion to a higher-paying, more responsible-sounding job. Notice the use of the term "more responsible-sounding." The last thing on any Overachieving Underperformer's wish list is more work to avoid doing.

Thankfully there are—especially in larger corporations—upper-management positions that require little to no actual work aside from attending meetings and conferences, and occasionally getting your assistant to file things. And therein lies the ultimate luxury of being an executive: The Personal Assistant.

The Hardworking Executive

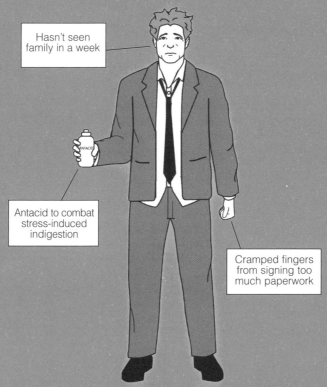

Hasn't seen family in a week

Antacid to combat stress-induced indigestion

Cramped fingers from signing too much paperwork

There's an unspoken truism in business: The less work actually required by executives, the more assistants they have working for them. Most senior corporate folk work on what they'll ominously refer to as "big picture" issues, implying that what goes on behind their closed doors are matters of such intellectual depth that only an elite class of business professionals could possibly

The Overachieving Underperforming Executive

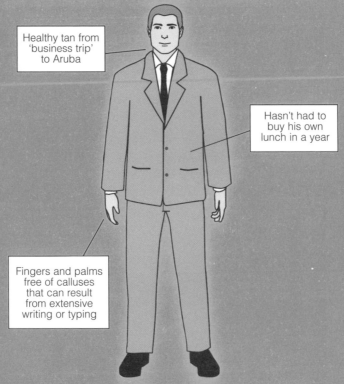

Healthy tan from 'business trip' to Aruba

Hasn't had to buy his own lunch in a year

Fingers and palms free of calluses that can result from extensive writing or typing

begin to understand. The truth is that most of these people spend their time on the phone talking to similarly positioned executives at other companies about when to meet for lunch. With the right person sitting outside your office door fielding phone calls and deflecting responsibility, you can go years without even knowing what your job is supposed to be.

Chapter 21

Judging the Poker Face:
Hints on Hiring

Once you've mastered the machinations and backstabbing required to get to a level where you're deemed worthy of a personal assistant, the most important thing is to hire the right type of assistant for your needs. Generally speaking, you will require above all else a good and tactful liar, someone who could not only convince Einstein that 2+2=5, but also make him regret ever having contested the issue.

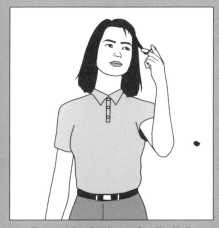

Be on the lookout for "tells" that could be potential giveaways when your assistant is lying for you, like hair twirling ...

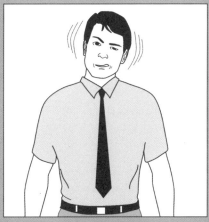

... or facial tics.

Like a good poker player, study your interview subject and watch for any "tells," physical signs such as chin scratching or looking off to the side, that indicate the speaker is being untruthful. If she keeps repeating the same tell, it won't be long before other people immediately pick up on her bluff. If she has multiple tics, you're dealing with a higher-caliber prevaricator and a potential employee. And if she can lie her way through an entire interview without broadcasting her bluffs, you shouldn't just hire her as your assistant, you should retain her as your tax attorney too. Here are some questions that you can ask to calibrate someone's capacity for mendacity.

 1 **"What were your grades like in college?"**
- Interviewee A: "I was a solid C/C-plus student."
- Interviewee B: "Mostly B-pluses, a few A-minuses."
- Interviewee C: "I made Dean's List every semester and graduated Phi Beta Kappa."

Analysis:
- Interviewee A: Do not hire. Much too honest and therefore of no use to you.
- Interviewee B: There's a chance that he may be telling you the truth; it's more likely, however, that he was a lazy student but is a decent liar. Continue with the interview.
- Interviewee C: He's either much too intelligent, studious, and ambitious to abide an Overachieving Underperformer like yourself, or he's a terrible fibber; either way, into the trash can with that résumé.

② "I really love that new movie *Disappearing Sunrise.* . . . Ever seen it?"

- Interviewee A: "No. Did you just make that up?"
- Interviewee B: "It sounds really familiar. Who's in it?"
- Interviewee C: "Oh my God! That scene with the elephant? Heartbreaking ..."

Analysis:

- Interviewee A: Again, this person's honesty is getting him nowhere. And yes, you did make it up.
- Interviewee B: A political, intelligent response; bonus points for putting it back on you for more information. This person would be good at deflecting unwanted phone calls and visitors.
- Interviewee C: He is either completely insane or he's got your number. Either way, a good assistant he would not make.

③ "Baroque Neoclassicism or Phenomenological Modernism?"

- Interviewee A: "I'm sorry ... Did you say something?"
- Interviewee B: "Well, that's really a matter of personal taste, and, while I have my preference, it would be unwise for me to say that one is actually better than the other."
- Interviewee C: "I live and die by the Seven Tenets of the DeStijl Movement."

Analysis:

- Interviewee A: Not even an attempt to fake his way through it. Just because you've no idea what someone's talking about doesn't mean you can't have a discussion on that topic. This person will crumple like tinfoil under the slightest pressure.

- Interviewee B: Perhaps a little too moderate an answer, but even if he's lying through his teeth, he could make you believe he's at least keeping pace with you.
- Interviewee C: Again, either too educated or completely overreaching in his attempt at deception.

4 *(Showing them a picture of a dog)* **"This is my daughter. Isn't she just precious?"**

- Interviewee A: "Um, that's a dog. You're making me uncomfortable."
- Interviewee B: "Wow ... You two must have a very special relationship."
- Interviewee C: "Is she single?"

Analysis:

- Interviewee A: This calls-'em-like-he-sees-'em rube has wasted enough of your time.
- Interviewee B: Again, tactful without being sycophantic. This person is your best choice.
- Interviewee C: The less said about this guy the better.

NOTE: You can create as many questions as you'd like, but keep in mind that you're looking for people who can talk themselves (and by extension, you) out of awkward situations. Thus, you want to find topics where the interviewee must either be honest or sidestep the issue completely.

Chapter 22

Follow My Lead:
The Coattails Effect

Next to a talent for stone-faced lying, the most important quality an Overachieving Underperformer requires in an assistant is an unflagging sense of loyalty. It's one thing to have someone lying to others and doing your work for you, but that will only last as long as the liar in question believes he's doing it for a good reason. You may luck out and happen upon someone who simply "gets it," but more than likely you'll need to nurture your assistant to foster a deep devotion.

Since most assistants take their entry-level positions in the hopes of achieving greater successes in the future, a tried and true method for developing dependency is to convince your assistant that you are destined for greatness and he or she is going along for the ride to the top. Whether or not you actually intend on piggybacking your assistant up the corporate ladder, here are some tips to help you keep that loyalty leash snug around your assistant's neck.

1. There's no "I" in "Team," but there is "Work" in "Teamwork"

The first move you must make with any assistant is to make him feel like he's fulfilling a crucial role in your life. For every phone call he screens, for every cup of coffee he retrieves, thank him; let him know that he's an outstanding employee and that you see brilliant things down the road for him if he keeps up like this.

Eventually, you'll begin passing along menial paperwork tasks to your assistant. Of course, if you're employed by a mammoth corporate entity, most of your work probably *is* menial paperwork. But there's no need for your assistant to know that he's now handling half your workload if he assumes it's only a small portion of your epically important job. And compared with the other assistants in the office, many of whose bosses yell at them for messing up the coffee and won't let them near any important papers, your assistant will be emboldened with a sense of worth and value, all thanks to you.

2. "Big Changes"

After gaining your assistant's trust and admiration, you'll need to drop hints to him that your next big promotion (and thus his) is virtually moments away. Drop whispered phrases into his ear like "I've heard some big changes are going to happen in the next couple months ..." and then smile, as if to imply that these changes will involve bigger and better things for you both. Take long lunches with friends, but tell your assistant something like "I can't say who exactly I'm meeting for lunch, but let's just say that GlobalCorp is looking for a new Senior VP ... and that Senior VP will need an assistant." Again, GlobalCorp may very well be looking for a new executive, but that has absolutely nothing to do with your lunch with your old college roommate. Your assistant, however, remains blissfully ignorant, dreaming of what to buy with his increased salary. In addition to being loyal to you, he'll cover for your extended afternoon away from the office.

3 Making Good

You can only have your assistant believing that you'll carry him on your able shoulders into the higher echelons of the corporation for so long until you have to show him something for his efforts. Of course, the best way to make good on empty promises is with empty actions:

a   Tell your assistant that he has been promoted from "Executive Assistant" to "Assistant Executive." Ask him not to be too vocal about his "promotion." Blame the secrecy on vaguely ominous "office politics." This will help make him slightly fearful that others are out to halt his rapid rise.

b   Get business cards printed up with the new title. If it costs you fifty dollars, it may be the best money you've ever spent so long as it keeps the assistant happy and away from the classified ads.

c   Invite your assistant along on every third business lunch. Why not? It's not as if you're paying. Be sure to introduce him as your "associate."

Chapter 23

"He's in a Meeting," or the Human "Do Not Disturb" Sign

As an executive, it's your company-given prerogative to close your door tight against the outside world whenever you wish. While you have free reign to barge into your subordinates' offices unannounced, your office is your "me space," your home away from home, and you are not to be interrupted. However, acting like that isn't going to help with your likability quotient, which is why it is a huge help to have someone else guarding the door. For those of you fortunate enough to have a personal assistant, you can have your cake, and you can eat it in privacy.

With your loyal assistant perched directly in front of your office door like some workplace sentry, it would be nearly impossible for someone to so much as knock on your door without permission. Thus, you can rest easy (heck, you can probably sleep if you want) in the knowledge that your nonworking will go undisturbed by anyone daring to bring you anything to sign or to look over.

For most visitors to your office, a simple "He's in a meeting" will suffice to turn them away, back to their desks. However, there are situations where persistent pests will not be shooed away so easily.

Problem Situation #1

The Scene: You're in the office talking on the telephone (personal call, long distance, of course) and you'd rather not be disturbed. But that's not going to stop a pesky Operations Manager from trying to interrupt your downtime. Luckily, you've hired a brilliant assistant.

Pest: "Steve in?"

Assistant: "He's in a meeting."

Pest: "But I can hear him through the door."

Assistant: "I said he's in a meeting."

Pest: "Then who is that I hear talking?"

Assistant: "The meeting is in his office."

Pest: "Why don't I hear any other voices?"

Assistant: "It's a conference call."

Pest: "That's not really a meeting!"

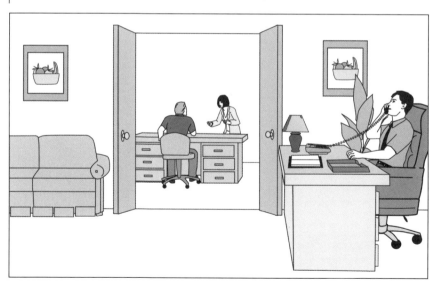

Assistant: "I'm not going to argue semantics with you. Please come back when he's off the phone."
Pest: "When will that be?"
Assistant: "Whenever the meeting is over."

At this point the conversation will either loop back into the discussion of the difference between a "meeting" and a "conference call," or the Pest will storm away in frustration. Either way, you've been able to book your flight to Fiji in peace and your assistant looks like the stubborn one.

Problem Situation #2

The Scene: You've just come back from a huge lunch (paid for by someone else, obviously), and you really need a nap if you're going to make it through that movie after work.

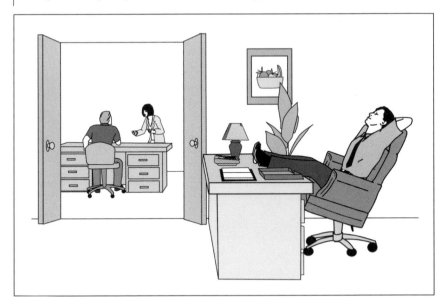

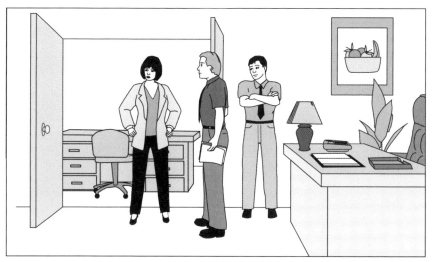

Pest: "I've just got to ask Steve a quick question."
Assistant: "He's in a meeting."
Pest: "But I just saw him walk in there!"
Assistant: "Who?"
Pest: "Steve!"
Assistant: "Oh, he's in a meeting. Can I just take a message?"
Pest: "But I know he's in there."
Assistant: "I doubt it ... Let me check." *(Assistant calls into the office, lets it ring twice and hangs up; this is a signal for Steve to get up and hide behind the door.)*
Assistant: "He's not answering. He must still be in that meeting."
Pest: "All right. Fine. If he's not in the office, can I just leave these papers on his desk?"
Assistant: "I'll take those. No need to clutter up his desk any more than it already is."

Pest: "Hah! You don't want me going in there!"

Assistant: "Would you like to watch me put them in his in-box?"

Problem Situation #3

The Scene: Your office is empty because you're out playing golf. But your assistant can't let the Pest know that.

Pest: "Where's Steve?"

Assistant: "He's in a meeting."

Pest: "Yeah, I know. You told me that two hours ago. I checked every conference room in the building and couldn't find him."

Assistant: "He's in a meeting in another office."

Pest: "You could have mentioned that!"

Assistant: "You didn't ask."

Pest: "What other office?"

Assistant: "I'm not sure. He left me a number where he could be reached."

Pest: "Give me the number; I need to talk to him."

Assistant: "I said he left *me* a number so *I* can reach him."

Pest: "Fine. Could you dial that number and ask him where those 400T Forms are?"

(Assistant dials Steve's cell phone number.)

Assistant *(into phone)*: "Yes, could I speak to Steve Johnson please? He's meeting with John Hemingway. Uh-huh? Okay, thanks. *(To Pest)*: They're in a meeting and they're not to be disturbed."

And once again, the Pest is defeated by deception, stubbornness, and circular logic, and all without interrupting your solid afternoon on the back nine.

Chapter 24

"Hold My Calls,"
or the Human Answering Machine

We live in an age when almost everyone has caller ID on mobile and home phones, allowing us to screen telemarketers, dodge ex-relations gone sour, and generally pick and choose to whom we will lend an ear. So why is it that many office phones don't also allow us to know who is on the other end waiting to annoy us before we pick up the receiver?

Even if you're fortunate enough to have caller ID on your office phone (many systems can only ID internal extensions and do nothing for calls from the outside world), it's almost more of an aggravation to have to sit inactive while waiting for your voice mail to kick in. This is especially true when confronted with a caller who knows full well that you're at your desk and just not answering. These irritating sorts will continue to hang up and try again until you ultimately cave under the constant ringing. Some phones have a "Do Not Disturb" function that automatically funnels incoming calls to your voice mail. However, what if you're waiting for your sister to call and tell you what your crazy uncle did at the family reunion? You certainly don't want to miss that.

But for the blessed executive, there exists an invention that answers the phone and screens calls at the same time, and it's the same personal assistant who covers for you while you're "in a meeting." If you so desire (and if you're reading this, you more than likely do), you'll not only never have to lift the receiver, you may never have to make a business call again.

 ## Making a List, Checking It Twice

Of course, your assistant is going to need to learn how to suss out the good (personal) callers from the bad (work-related) callers. You'll need to familiarize your assistant with who is and isn't welcome. The best way to do this is in list form.

Since it's better to be safe than caught in a conversation with your VP of Fulfillment, the first list your assistant will require is the "I'm not here" group—those folks who only have unpleasant things to say and who also have a tendency to drone on ad nauseam about them.

Your assistant has a prepared list of things to say to these dreary souls. For example:
"She's in a meeting. Can I take a message?" (See Chapter 23)
"He's on a call with [fill in name of feared senior executive]. Can I take a message?"
"He's not taking any calls from anyone right now. Can I take a message?"
"She's in the bathroom. Can I take a message?
"She just stepped out. Can I take a message? No, she didn't say where. Can I take a message?"

NOTE: As you may have picked up on, it's of the utmost importance for your assistant to get to the "Can I take a message?" portion of the phone call, this being the fastest way to get rid of an annoying caller.

Eventually, after taking many messages and waylaying many visitors for you, your assistant will develop a solid grasp of what you're supposed to be working on. As this happens you'll be able to simply dictate a return message to the assistant, who will then make the call, relieving you of even more responsibility.

Overachieving at Underperforming

With a savvy enough assistant, you'll be left completely out of the loop on business calls and your assistant will be doing your job for (and probably better than) you. And when someone takes you to task for not knowing all the fine details of your work, you reply, simply, "My assistant deals with the details. I'm thinking Big Picture."

② With Friends Like These . . .

You'll also need to provide your assistant with a roster of all your friends and family (or at least those to whom you wish to occasionally speak). These should be sorted in some sort of priority.

 It's recommended that you keep your friends and family list in an easily altered electronic form such as a spreadsheet or database. These formats allow you to clearly color-code individuals and rearrange priorities at will, depending on your mood or the time of year.

Interns:
The Best Things in Life Are Free

Just because you haven't reached the rung on the executive ladder that merits you an assistant doesn't mean you can't find someone to treat like one. Every summer hordes of college students flood the corporate landscape in a veritable tsunami of free labor. Inexperienced, naïve, and possibly educated, these youngsters are begging to be exploited by anyone with a business card.

1 **Getting an Intern**

Depending on your particular position, there are varying degrees of difficulty in acquiring an intern. Consider two scenarios:

- If your company doesn't normally have interns, it shouldn't be too hard to convince your boss that some free labor could be helpful. (After all, just look at how early you've been having to come in!)
- Oddly enough, in a corporate setting where interns are a given, it can often require considerable legwork to get one of these unwitting undergrads for yourself. Here, the layers of corporate bureaucracy that are your friends when it comes to obscuring your inefficiency are turned against you; you must navigate them with stealth in order to convince the appropriate parties that,

WARNING: Nepotism is your enemy. Many interns are related to someone you work with, and it's usually someone much more important than you. Do whatever you can to avoid getting stuck with the VP's pudding-brained nephew. Generally speaking, these interns are much less likely to do any of your work and much more likely to rat you out if it might get themselves a pat on the back.

indeed, you could use some serious intern assistance. It will help your case if, in the period of time immediately leading up to the influx of interns, you amp up the level of clutter in your office. If your boss should fail to comment, be proactive and apologize to her for the mess; you've just been *so* busy recently. If only you had some help ...

2 Keeping the Intern and Acquiring More

- As soon as you're able to nail down some free help, you'll want to train him in every possible detail of your job (or at least the ones you haven't already been able to dole out indefinitely to others).
- Make him believe that this is a once-in-a-lifetime opportunity that will give him a huge leg up on the competition after graduating. Remind him repeatedly of the letter of recommendation that you'll write when this is all through.
- Compliments are always the easiest way to keep someone on your side. Tell him, "It's a shame you've got to go back to school. You're ready for the real world now." And, "You've got a better handle on the business than most of the salaried people here!"
- Don't be an intern hog. Occasionally rent out your intern to your less-kind coworkers, especially for their most menial and mind-numbing tasks. Your temporary assistant will come running back to you, ready to complete and file paperwork.
- When your intern's tenure is up, make sure he has done a magnificent job of cleaning up your work area, then assume an air that is (slightly) happier and (a little) less frazzled. As your office reverts to its typically chaotic state mere hours after your intern checks out on his final day, you'll once again receive pitying glances from your higher-ups. Put on an Oscar-worthy performance and you'll be earmarked for *two* interns when next summer rolls around.

Chapter 25

When the Cat's Away: Making Your Assistant Glad That You're Out of the Office

Even though the focus thus far has been on playing the part of a "good boss" and on showing your assistant a great deal of generosity, there is still something to be said for occasionally being an unpleasant person to work for. If your boss-assistant relationship is too familiar, your assistant might begin to think that he or she can take advantage of the situation and start to emulate your nonworking habits. Behavior such as this needs to be nipped in the bud. Here are some potential problem situations with suggested solutions.

Coming In Late

Situation: Noticing that you don't usually arrive until well after ten a.m., your assistant's arrival time begins to slacken until she's arriving mere moments before you do. (You can tell because you used to do the same thing and can recognize the signs.)

Solution: Make an effort one morning to actually arrive at the office on time. But instead of going into your office, sit at your assistant's desk and wait for her arrival. When she does arrive, don't get angry. Merely act disappointed and say, "I figured since you weren't here to do your job, I might as well do it." Let the words hang in the air for a few moments before going into your office for a nap.

TIP *This works even better if you can manage to arrange for someone to call you while you're chiding your assistant. Don't let her answer the phone. Instead, answer it and refer to yourself in the third person, pretending to be your own assistant.*

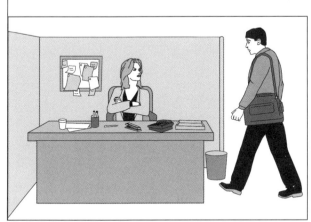

"I figured since you weren't here to do your job, I might as well do it."

Result: Your assistant will be on time for at least the next month, and she'll be so embarrassed at having been caught that she will not only cover for you when you disappear for the entire afternoon, but also thank you for disappearing.

2 Getting Too Personal

Situation: Your assistant's view of you begins to change from "boss" to "buddy." Before you know it, she might begin asking for favors or wasting your time with her personal issues, when you'd much rather be wasting your time on *your* personal issues.

Solution: The next time your assistant comes to you in a chitchatty mood, babbling on about some awful date she'd been on or some other nonsense, look at her sternly and ask, "Do you think this is really an appropriate conversation to be having with a coworker?"

Result: Your assistant will avoid any unnecessary conversation for a few days, which means she won't be paying too much attention to your comings and goings, nor will she dare to ask prying questions when she overhears you having personal phone conversations. Additionally, this period of awkward tension gives you a chance to load her up with busy work. All this will make it a great six hours for her when you don't come into the office until the late afternoon next Monday.

3 Ego Check

Situation: The assistant has gotten over all her first-job growing pains and is starting to get a bit smug about how quickly and efficiently she does her (your) job. If you don't knock her down a peg, she could start looking elsewhere for a better job.

Solution: Stay late one night and empty some old filing cabinets. Shuffle up the files so that nothing is where it should be. Leave them in piles of assorted sizes and types all over her work space so that she sees everything as soon as she comes within view of her desk. When she asks you what's going on, quickly put on your coat and say, "I spent all morning looking for those McCool papers. I had to pull all of these files, and still nothing. Now I've got to go and deal with this situation in person. You *must* be more careful when filing things away. Make sure these all get put back before I return." Then leave without any further explanation. Your assistant will be sent into a tizzy trying to figure out what she did to disappoint you, where these papers belong, and just how long she has before you get back. She'll figure it all out soon enough, and she'll be happy that you were gone until four thirty.

TIP *If you really want to rub it in, wait until your assistant is gone that day and pull everything back out. When she comes in the next morning, repeat the previous day's statement as you leave, adding, "And be more careful this time; these were all out of order." This way, not only can you vanish for the whole day, but the next morning is a safe bet too.*

Chapter 26

Need-to-Know: Why You Should Never Tell Your Assistant the Whole Truth

The truth is often much less interesting, and less useful (for your purposes) than offering selected tidbits of information. What's the use of telling your assistant the entire story when feeding him little slices gets him to do what you want? Here are some examples where the reality of the situation would never get the results achieved with edited half-truths.

1 The Budget Slash

You say: "I've heard they're going to slash the department's budget by thirty percent."

What your assistant hears: "We'd better straighten up and fly right or else we might get the ax."

What you're not saying: The "department" in question is the city's sanitation department.

What you earn: An assistant who cuts down on the personal phone calls and will do whatever you put on his desk.

2 The Junior Executive

You say: "The management trainee group has asked me to nominate one junior-level employee."

What your assistant hears: "I really believe in you and want to help your career."

What you're not saying: That you've already nominated that cute assistant over in Accounts Payable.

What you earn: Until he realizes that he was not selected for the program, your assistant will work twelve hours a day and wash and wax your car if you ask. After he finds out, he'll look to you for solace and guidance. Tell him that his nomination was left out when the program was downsized, but that you'll definitely get him in next year.

3 Bound for Glory

You say: "The CEO and I were talking about you at the meeting yesterday."

What your assistant hears: "You're so destined for stardom, the bigwigs already know about you."

What you're not saying: That the only reason your assistant's name was mentioned to the CEO was because she asked you for the name of a good babysitter.

What you earn: An assistant who truly believes that you are looking out for his best interests. More importantly, an assistant who will do nothing to annoy you for fear that you would immediately cease dropping his name to other executives.

NOTE: Don't be afraid to offer up complete misinformation. That way, when the assistants all go out after work to drink away their small wages and compare notes, yours will have information that no one else could ... because it's entirely false.

4 Impending Doom

You say: "I was a little let down by your report on those quarterly figures."

What your assistant hears: "One more screwup and you're gone!"

What you're not saying: That the reason you feel "let down" is because the work was so much better than anything you would have done.

What you earn: An assistant who is worried for his job and who will now do even more work to impress you and get back into your good graces.

Chapter 27

A Rolling Assistant Gathers No Moss:
Why It's Good to Have Your Assistant Running Errands

Just as you sometimes need to play the tough boss so your assistant will be happy to have you out of his or her hair for a few hours (see Chapter 25), it's also a good idea to have your assistant occasionally away from the office for good chunks of time. Not only will it be good for her to get fresh air and see some daylight, but also it gives you time to do things that you'd otherwise not do while she's around. Here are some examples of the variety of chores and errands you can send your assistant out of the office to pursue:

1 Office Supplies

Task: Most large offices have managers whose entire job is to see that every department is fully stocked with all practical office equipment. And when something is required, it's usually ordered in bulk through a catalog. However, there are always certain items that either do not fall under the canon of Standard Office Supplies (protractors, slide rules, laser levels) or are needed right now, and these are what you dispatch your assistant out into the streets for. Don't be afraid to get creative with your requests. If you have an expense account to charge these items to, all the better.

Actual amount of time required: Thirty to forty-five minutes.

Allowable amount of time away from office: Approximately one hour.

Why this is good for your assistant: Aside from the guaranteed fifteen to thirty minutes of personal time she'll get, she knows that you'll be delighted that she was able to find *just* the right type of blue ballpoint pen for you.

What you can do in the time allotted: Quickly scan through your assistant's e-mails to see what she's been writing about you.

2 Anniversary/Birthday Gift

Task: You've got an occasion coming up where a gift is required, but you don't care enough about the recipient to go out and select a present yourself. So send your assistant out to the mall entrusted with your credit card and a fifty dollar budget, and she will surely find something nice.

Actual amount of time required: One hour maximum.

Allowable amount of time away from office: Up to two hours.

Why this is good for your assistant: You've shown a wealth of trust in her, both by giving her your personal credit card, and by allowing her carte blanche to select a proper gift.

What you can do in the time allotted: Watch a DVD on your computer.

3 Prescription Refills

Task: Your allergy medicine is running low. Send the assistant to pick it up.

Actual amount of time required: Fifteen to thirty minutes.

Allowable amount of time away from office: Up to ninety minutes.

Why this is good for your assistant: You show not only that you think of her as a reliable person but that you're open enough with her to share what medicines you take. She'll also enjoy ample free time while waiting for the prescription to be filled.

What you can do in the time allotted: Get a solid nap in before your three martini lunch.

4 Automobile Inspections/Repairs

Task: Your car needs an oil change every three thousand miles and its emissions inspected annually. Why waste your time taking the car yourself when you can waste your assistant's time and she'll be glad to do it?

Actual amount of time required: Forty-five to ninety minutes.

Allowable amount of time away from office: Ninety minutes to two hours.

Why this is good for your assistant: Being that you probably earn several times more than your assistant, you should certainly have a better car than she does. So at the very least, she will enjoy the chance to tool around town playing with the automatic car seats.

What you can do in the time allotted: Go out to lunch, come back. And then go out again as soon as she returns with your car.

5 **Wild Goose Chase**

Task: You don't necessarily need a task to get your assistant away for a few hours. With a little help from your friends, you can have your assistant ping-ponging back and forth across the city for an entire afternoon.

Tell your assistant that she has to go over to another office and get some papers from a guy named Mark (a childhood friend). When she arrives at Mark's office, she'll be told that she was given the wrong information and that she needs to go downtown to another office and speak to Susan (another friend) who will in turn say that she just messengered the papers back up to Mark. With enough friends willing to have a good laugh, your assistant will spend more time on the road than she will at her desk.

Actual amount of time required: As much as a full day.

Allowable amount of time away from office: So long as you're not in danger of your assistant not getting your work done on time, it's up to you.

Why this is good for your assistant: It's not, really, but it's a lot of fun for you.

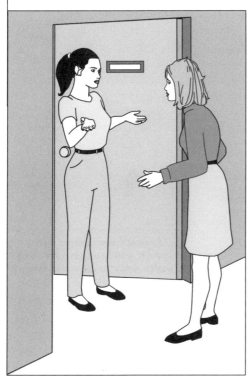

What you can do in the time allotted: Write a book about abusing the corporate system for your own enjoyment and financial betterment.

A Wild Goose Chase can keep an assistant out of your hair for up to one full day.

Giving Out Gold Stars:
Cheap Ways to Make Your Staff Happy

As a boss, you'll learn quickly that while some of your employees are only interested in financial and material gain, most are more than satisfied with being shown that they are appreciated. So, instead of giving your employees the pay raise they deserve, use any of the following methods to keep them satisfied with the status quo.

 Candy

It's a rare person who is not a fan of sweets. Scour the sale racks at your local grocery store and then shower your employees with sugar and chocolate.
Cost: Less than ten dollars.
Effect: Even the rare person who avoids candy will see the gesture in a

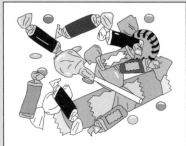

Sweets and candy are a quick and inexpensive way to make your employees happy.

positive light. You will be viewed as a cool, generous boss who likes to keep his workers happy and who is in touch with their wants and needs.
Duration: Until the sweets disappear; two hours at the most.

2 **Notes/Cards**

For some reason, a handwritten note—regardless of content— is taken to mean much more than something typed or sent by e-mail. And when that note says something nice, it's that much more moving. So the next time you get a bonus for something your assistant wrote for you, leave a really nice note written out on a card.

Cost: Less than five dollars.

Effect: The receiver will be flattered and impressed with your gratitude. You might even receive a thank-you card in return.

Duration: Up to one week.

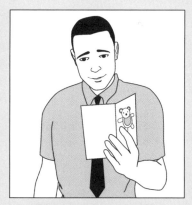

Many assistants will so value cards expressing a boss's gratitude that they will actually keep them.

3 **Lunch**

As an executive, you've either got people constantly taking you out to lunch or you're returning the favor and using your expense account to pay for the meal. Chances are your employees are not so lucky and must always pay for their modest midday meals. Instead of promoting a good employee, invite him along for a fancy lunch.

Cost: Free!

Effect: Should impress your employee enough to make him work even harder in hopes of being invited to future lunches.

Duration: About two to three weeks.

4 **Implied Promotions**

Executives often find themselves stuck on any number of useless committees and task forces that meet monthly and ultimately do nothing. Make one of your employees feel appreciated by sending him as your substitute to one of these groups.

Cost: Free!

Effect: The employee will view this as a sign of having your confidence, making him even more committed to your shared success, lest he disappoint you.

Duration: Up to six months, depending on how quickly the employee realizes that he's not getting a promotion out of this.

5 Frequent Flier Miles

If your senior position requires a good deal of travel, you may have racked up more frequent flier miles than you will ever have the chance to use. When you feel that one of your workers is becoming unhappy, offer her a free round-trip ticket anywhere in the country.

Cost: Free!

Effect: Regardless of the fact that you're not spending any of your money, your employees will view this gesture as you reaching into your own pocket and paying for the vacation yourself. Devotion above and beyond the call of duty will ensue.

Duration: About a year (until the next year comes around and you don't make the same offer).

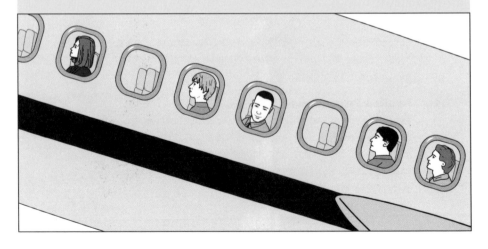

There it goes again: your alarm. In another time, a lesser you would have slumped out of bed and raced to join the rush to work. But you know better now. And so you hit the snooze button and return to your gentle slumber. When eventually you do rise from bed, you linger at the window while calmly enjoying breakfast, peering out with curiosity at folks running to catch a train or stuck in commuter traffic. You find it hard to believe that you were once like them.

The situation is similar when you finally make your way in to work. Others scurry around frantically while you calmly nap behind the closed door of your office, or you disappear for hours on end to go shopping or catch an afternoon matinee. From the moment of your late arrival until your audaciously early departure a few hours later, you'll be paid to do nothing. And they'll love you for it.

But remember, the lessons you've learned are only as good as their application. Like any complex machine, being an Overachieving Underperformer requires constant maintenance and supervision. If you lapse into laziness and lose focus on your idleness for even a short period, it won't be a far walk to the unemployment line. But for those willing to work hard at hardly working, there's no limit to how far you can let other people's work take you.

Chris Morran has hardly worked for numerous major publishing and advertising companies. He's also an award-winning playwright, actor, and comic who has written and performed for the Upright Citizens Brigade Theatre and the Yankee Rep Theatre Co. He lives in New York City.